Contemporary Ayurveda

Pg 7 – words for M A V = Maharishi ayur Veda

Exercise – regular in Moderation.

D1429952

Contemporary Ayurveda
Medicine and Research in Maharishi Ayur-Veda

Hari Sharma MD FRCPC

Professor Emeritus and Former Director, Cancer Prevention and Natural Products Research, Department of Pathology, College of Medicine, The Ohio State University, Columbus, Ohio, USA; Fellow, National Academy of Ayurveda, Ministry of Health and Family Welfare, Government of India, India

Christopher Clark MD

Medical Director, Maharishi Ayur-Veda Health Center, Raj Health Resort, Fairfield, Iowa, USA; Founding Faculty and Assistant Clinical Professor of Physiology, College of Maharishi Vedic Medicine, Maharishi University of Management, Fairfield, Iowa, USA

Foreword by

Gary Kaplan MD PhD

Director of Clinical Neurophysiology, North Shore University Hospital, Associate Professor of Clinical Neurology, New York University School of Medicine, New York, USA

Series Editor

Marc Micozzi MD PhD

Executive Director, College of Physicians, Philadelphia, Pennsylvania, USA; Adjunct Professor, Department of Rehabilitation Medicine, University of Pennsylvania School of Medicine, Philadelphia, Pennsylvania, USA

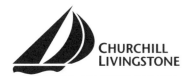

CHURCHILL
LIVINGSTONE

EDINBURGH LONDON PHILADELPHIA TOKYO

CHURCHILL LIVINGSTONE
A Harcourt Health Sciences Company

The rights of Hari Sharma and Christopher Clark to be
identified as the authors of this Work have been asserted by
them in accordance with the Copyright, Designs, and Patents
Act 1988.

First published 1998
    Fourth impression 2001

ISBN 0 443 05594 7

British Library Cataloguing in Publication Data
A catalogue record for this book is available from the British
Library.

Library of Congress Cataloging in Publication Data
A catalog record for this book is available from the Library of
Congress.

Note
Medical knowledge is constantly changing. As new
information becomes available, changes in treatment,
procedures, equipment and the use of drugs become
necessary. The authors and the publishers have, as far as it is
possible, taken care to ensure that the information given in
this text is accurate and up-to-date. However, readers are
strongly advised to confirm that the information, especially
with regard to drug usage, complies with latest legislation
and standards of practice.

Printed in China
SWTC/04

Contents

Introduction to the Series

The aim of this Series is to provide, for health care professionals and students, clear and rational guides to what is currently known about:

- therapeutic medical systems currently labeled as complementary medicine
- complementary approaches to specific medical conditions
- integration of complementary therapy into mainstream medical practice.

Each text is written specifically with the needs and questions of a health care audience in mind. Where possible, basic applications in clinical practice are explored.

What is called complementary medicine is being rapidly integrated into mainstream health care largely in response to consumer demand, but also, in recognition of new scientific findings that are expanding our view of health and healing – and pushing against the limits of the current biomedical paradigm.

Health care professionals need to know what their patients are doing and what they believe about what has been called alternative medicine. In addition, a basic working knowledge of complementary medical therapies is a rapidly growing requirement for primary care, some medical specialties, and throughout the allied health professions. These approaches also expand our view of the art and science of medicine and contribute importantly to the intellectual formation of health professions students.

This Series provides a survey of the fundamentals and foundations of complementary medical systems currently available and practiced in North America and Europe. Each topic is presented in ways that are *understandable* and that provide an important *understanding* of the intellectual foundations of each system – with translation between the complementary and conventional medical systems, where possible. These explanations draw appropriately on the social and scientific foundations of each system of care.

Rapidly growing contemporary research results are included whenever possible. In addition to providing evidence indicating where complementary medicines may be of therapeutic benefit, guidance is provided as to when complementary therapies should not be used, as well.

This field of health is rapidly moving from being considered *alternative* (implying exclusive use of one medical system or another), to *complementary* (used as an adjunct to mainstream medical care), to *integrative medicine* (implying an active, conscious effort by mainstream medicine to incorporate alternatives on the basis of rational clinical and scientific information and judgment).

Likewise, health care professionals and students must move rapidly to learn the fundamentals of complementary medical systems in order to better serve their patients' needs, protect the public health, and expand their scientific horizons and understandings of health and healing.

1997   Marc S. Micozzi

Foreword

In years to come, the 20th century will no doubt be referred to as the century of science and technology. The great expansion of these fields paved the way for the development of modern medicine. The success of the modern medical approach is based on its ability to use the scientific method to clarify in ever greater detail the symptoms and signs of specific diseases, and to develop potent medications for the alleviation of some of those signs and symptoms, often aiding in the removal of the disease itself. This approach has met with success because, being science-based, it allows us to evaluate objectively which treatments work and which do not. In addition, expanding technology has given us new and very powerful tools to aid in diagnosis, and at times to alter manifestations of disease states.

However, as grateful as we are as physicians for the benefits of modern medicine, we may sometimes collectively feel that we have not created a truly healthy society. The greatest advances in health in this century have come about because of improved sanitation, not because of new medications or surgical techniques. We are still plagued by new and more virulent infectious diseases, though our antibiotic armamentarium is stronger than it has ever been. Atherosclerotic diseases including myocardial infarction and stroke persist in their high prevalence, though we can alter their course with medication and surgery. The same is true for a myriad of cancers.

Our efforts to decrease the incidence of these diseases, and prolong survival with such illnesses, have been aided by the use of modern medical techniques, which are often associated with unacceptable side-effects. Such side-effects range from minor, though potentially disabling, sedation and dizziness to more serious complications such as hemorrhage, convulsions, antibiotic resistance, or the induction of a new malignancy as a result of therapy to treat a prior malignancy.

What is needed is a new approach, an approach that will prevent disease by strengthening normal physiologic functions at all levels. This approach should promote health at each level of the human organism, from the subtle field of molecular interaction, through the levels of cellular function and organ system function, to the physiologic functioning of the whole individual. If a new approach is worthwhile, its effects on promoting health should be measurable at each of these levels. We need not accept serious health risks and side-effects as unavoidable features of health care.

It is not enough to say that the current system has often failed us, and that a new approach is needed. A new approach to health must meet stringent criteria to gain acceptance in the medical community. That approach must have solid theoretical and experimental foundations which provide a unique and profound understanding of the physical and biological laws which govern human physiology. If such an understanding is not present, or is not scientifically verifiable, then the 'new approach' is just another in the vast group of alternative medicines, appealing to some, but unlikely to significantly affect the health of individuals or their community.

A revival of Ayurveda known as Maharishi Ayur-Veda, described in this volume, has attempted to meet the criteria set forth above. Evidence of its theoretical and experimental foundations is presented, and it is possible to see that simple and natural techniques have positive effects on health which may be objectively verified. Moreover, the authors present a new framework for our understanding of health and the cause of disease. This framework provides a different model for understanding the relations of individual health with the whole of nature – a model that has, as the authors show, possible parallels with advanced theories of quantum physics. The premise of Maharishi Ayur-Veda is to take modern medicine from the age of increasingly sophisticated anatomical, physiological, biochemical, and molecular manipulations to an age of technologies of the unified field. Drs Sharma and Clark have provided clear guideposts for this journey.

1996   Gary P. Kaplan

Preface

Health care in the contemporary political entity of the state of India is a heterogeneous mix drawing on the medical traditions of both Asia and Europe as a legacy of its own history. Various medical systems and traditions are officially sanctioned and supported by the state.

The 'original' medical tradition of the cultures indigenous to present-day India drew on Ayurveda, 'the way of life', or the 'science of life, or longevity'. At once more and less than a medical system per se, Ayurveda is a prescription for living (with many proscriptions as well). From this philosophy of life derived from ancient teachings and wisdom a medical system can be articulated. As a somewhat 'loosely' organized set of traditions, the medical aspects of Ayurveda may be highly *individuated* among 'patients' and practitioners, and to some extent the line between what allopathic medicine might traditionally consider a patient versus a practitioner is somewhat blurred.

During successive occupations of India by Islamic, and then European rulers, the traditions of Ayurveda were lost or actively suppressed, and other medical traditions were introduced. To the extent that Ayurveda ever represented an integrated system, it became somewhat disintegrated. Contemporary Ayurveda as treated in this text represents a conscious attempt to revive and reconstruct some principles and practices of Ayurveda (a kind of cultural 'revival' or restoration), to present it as an integrated system and to interpret it in the light of some contemporary theories of fundamental science that reach beyond Newtonian mechanics and typological biology (what I have called 'pre-Darwinian biology') as an explanation of health.

This particular system of Ayurveda is a fully articulated system that is manifest in its theoretical constructs, body of knowledge, training, and practice and is increasingly available in providing clinical services in North America. The system described in this text has made a conscious effort to consider the culture and society of contemporary North America in designing and delivering the type of health care described.

Therefore, this text provides a representation of how Ayurveda as a medical system may be encountered in North America and Europe today. Other Ayurvedic traditions are also encountered in the US today, but are generally not integrated in the manner described above. In India, individual traditions of Ayurveda still flourish alongside Islamic medical traditions, homeopathy (introduced by European physicians during the last century) and allopathic medicine as found in contemporary North America and Europe. It is hard to say which system is dominant in India, and the political state makes no such distinction. The Indian population freely picks and chooses from among different medical traditions depending upon their needs and the availability of resources. This heterogeneous mix serves the second largest national population in the world.

This may be a reflection of the recognition that allopathic medicine is neither an appropriate nor an affordable medical technology for many situations. Another view may suggest that the present situation in India is associated with a lower standard of medical care. The historical antecedents of the present-day health and nutritional status of the Indian population may be discussed and debated with respect to the role of European contact; the net result is a health-care system which actively draws on both Asian and European traditions as a kind of 'popular medicine' in India, and which has provided the basis for a contemporary system that is widely available and increasingly popular in North America.

1996   Marc S. Micozzi

Acknowledgments

We would like first to express our deepest appreciation to Maharishi Mahesh Yogi for imparting his knowledge of consciousness and of Ayurveda.

Next, we wish to thank our families, for their constant love, patience, and support.

We would also like to thank the pre-eminent Ayurvedic *vaidyas* who have so generously shared their vast knowledge of Ayurveda with us, in particular Dr Brihaspati Dev Triguna, Dr Balraj Maharshi, the late Dr V. M. Dwivedi, Dr H. S. Kasture, Dr P. D. Subedhar, Dr Jaya Ramanuja Raju, and Dr Manohar Palakurthi. We also are grateful to the hundreds of physicians trained in Maharishi Ayur-Veda for their help in bringing out this knowledge. In particular, we wish to thank those leaders and initial proponents of Maharishi Ayur-Veda in the USA, Drs Richard Averbach and Stuart Rothenberg, for their pioneering efforts and for the knowledge they have made available to so many; Dr Tony Nader for his landmark discoveries about the connections of Vedic literature and the physiology; and Dr Barry Charles for his tireless efforts on behalf of Maharishi Ayur-Veda.

Finally, we are grateful to Barney Sherman and Robert and Patricia Oates for their editorial assistance, and Linda Egenes and Ellen Kauffman for their research assistance.

H. S., C. C.

Dedicated to Maharishi Mahesh Yogi

Introduction: What Maharishi Ayur-Veda offers to clinical medicine

Maharishi Ayur-Veda (MAV) is a systematically developed, carefully researched medical system based on the ancient Indian medical system known as Ayurveda. The word '*ayurveda*' means literally the knowledge or science (*veda*)* of life (*ayu*). Ayurveda's exact age is not known, but stretches back several millennia. Ancient Vedic texts describe its origins in a story about a convocation of *rishis* (enlightened sages). Concerned about increased ill health in the world, the *rishis* sought to uncover the deepest truths of human physiology and health so that something could be done to prevent or ease the suffering. To help attain this goal, they meditated together in a large group, while one of them, Bharadwaja, attempted to seek the answer. In the intensely coherent atmosphere created by the powerful minds of all meditating together, Bharadwaja cognized the essence of Ayurveda. The story conveys something of that essence. For one thing, as we will see in our final chapter, the concern with collective (population) health remains central in MAV. For another, the value of refining one's consciousness through meditation plays a fundamental role in MAV, as by all accounts it did in ancient Ayurveda.

Ayurveda was clearly a sophisticated system. Ancient Ayurvedic texts described blood circulation thousands of years before William Harvey described it in the West in the 17th century. They distinguished two types of diabetes. They identified the layers of the skin, and described surgical procedures and tools still used by contemporary medicine. Yet the conceptual

---

*See the Appendix at the end of the book for the pronunciation of Sanskrit words.

framework of these texts differs profoundly from that which guides contemporary biomedicine: as we said, it focuses on creating positive health as well as treating disease, and – as we will see in Chapter 2 – emphasizes the role of consciousness in creating health, an issue that Western medicine is only beginning to address.

Ayurveda was suppressed during the long periods of foreign rule in India. During centuries of colonial rule, Ayurvedic institutions were not officially supported and often, in fact, were actively suppressed. Much important clinical and theoretical knowledge was lost. Experts in the various approaches of Ayurveda – specialists in herbal medicines, purification procedures, diagnosis, and many other modalities – lost contact with each other and even began to conflict with one another. Most significantly, the central role of consciousness, of meditation and other mental techniques, was temporarily eclipsed.

When India became politically independent in 1947, Ayurveda was in disarray, with widely varying standards of quality and conflicts of opinion. A new spirit of national pride stimulated its revival. In 1971, Ayurveda was made part of India's official state healthcare system, which had until then been exclusively Western. Still, Ayurvedic experts felt that Ayurveda was not what it once had been. Some areas of Ayurveda recorded in ancient texts were essentially unavailable. The idea expressed above about consciousness and its applications to health was at most given lip-service. More important, in actual practise, Ayurveda had lost some of its preventive potency; it often amounted to only the dispensing of herbal medicines, which fell short of what most Ayurvedic experts sought. Some Ayurvedic experts accomplished a great deal; but some of the finest of them felt that Ayurveda had more potential than was yet fully realized.

When Maharishi Mahesh Yogi turned his attention to Ayurveda, his stated goal was to revive the system in its comprehensive and integrated form – with the help of the leading *vaidyas* (Ayurvedic physicians) of our time, and in accordance with the classical texts. More especially, his intent was to restore the role of consciousness to its central position, both theoretically and through practical techniques.

Maharishi, after receiving his knowledge from his master, Swami Brahmananda Saraswati, the Jagadguru Shankaracharya of Jyotir Math, has devoted almost 40 years to bringing ancient Vedic knowledge to the world, and to integrating that knowledge with Western science. He systematized the teaching of meditation, allowing him to train thousands of other people to give instruction in Transcendental Meditation (TM), which has now been learned by over 3 million people worldwide. He encouraged objective research on subjective meditation techniques. Hundreds of published studies clearly indicate that the mental and physical approaches he advocates are highly effective (Ch. 3). Further, he has worked extensively to detail the mechanics of intelligence – in nature and in the human mind – and to align these understandings with profound discoveries of scientific theory. Rather than pitting subjective and objective approaches against one another, he has led a unification of the two that he calls 'Vedic Science'. Finally, he has founded universities (such as Maharishi University of Management in the United States, and Maharishi Vedic Universities in many countries around the world) that teach all disciplines in the light of this integrated understanding of life.

In the early 1980s, Maharishi asked several leading *vaidyas* (Ayurvedic physicians) to collaborate with him in restoring Ayurveda to its full value. Maharishi's main collaborators were Dr B. D. Triguna, the late Dr V. M. Dwivedi, and Dr Balraj Maharshi. Dr Triguna is the former president of the All-India Ayurvedic Congress, the Ayurvedic equivalent of the AMA, and Director of the National Academy for Ayurveda. Triguna is also generally regarded as the foremost expert on Ayurvedic pulse diagnosis. Dr Dwivedi, a member of the Indian Government's Central Council on Indian Medicine, was recognized as a leader in Ayurveda's most important herbal preparations, called 'rasayanas'. Dr Balraj Maharshi, adviser on Ayurveda to the Government of Andhra Pradesh (a state in India), is considered unsurpassed in his knowledge of Ayurveda's materia medica. They were joined by other *vaidyas*, as well as by scholars, scientists, and Western physicians.

The result of this collaboration is now being practiced in clinics worldwide, including India, Europe, Japan, Africa, Russia, Australia, and South and North America, by MDs specially trained in MAV, many of whom also practice privately. MAV has several claims on medical attention. For one thing, it is the only approach to Ayurveda that has given rise to a surprisingly large body of published scientific research, whose results are often remarkable. Over 500 studies, conducted at research institutions around the world, have been published, mostly on consciousness modalities (especially TM) and on herbal supplements. For another, MAV has a profound theoretical basis. Finally, its practical applications in clinical settings around the world are proving effective.

THE NEED FOR A NEW MODEL

Another claim MAV has on medical attention is that it addresses certain problems within Western medicine itself. These are becoming more evident and are being brought up by mainstream physicians. 'We should make people aware of the uncertainties of medicine,' said Dr Roy Schwarz. 'Not everybody will be cured and in some cases disaster will occur. That's reality.' Medical practice, by necessity, he continued, always will be based on trial and error (Friend 1995). Dr Schwarz was the Vice-President for Scientific Education and Practice Standards for the American Medical Association. What he describes is something every experienced clinician knows.

The potential pitfalls are numerous. Consider iatrogenic (physician-caused) diseases, which some feel have reached epidemic proportions (Robin 1987). In the *Journal of the American Medical Association*, Dr Lucien Leape of Harvard School of Public Health reported that '180 000 people die in the US each year partly as a result of iatrogenic injury, the equivalent of three jumbo-jet crashes every two days' (Leape 1994). Another *JAMA* article noted that fatal injury from medical treatment in the US 'dwarfs the annual automobile accident mortality of 45 000 and accounts for more deaths than all other accidents combined' (Bates et al 1995). Hospitals are especially conducive to iatrogenic disease and injury: conservative, carefully controlled studies have found iatrogenic disease to afflict 36% of hospitalized patients, with up to a quarter of it being serious or fatal (Steel et al 1981, Brennan et al 1991). Aside from the grief that results, medicine-caused disorders cost the US economy tens of billions of dollars – about $76 billion in 1995 (Johnson & Bootman 1995).

A related problem – and part of the reason for what one doctor called the 'iatroepidemic' – is that Western treatments of consequence usually produce side-effects. Much of this has to do with the central treatment modality of medicine, the drug. 2 to 5% of patients admitted to medical and pediatric services of general hospitals are there because of illnesses 'attributed to drugs' (Isselbacher et al 1994). Studies have found that up to half of iatrogenic injuries in hospitals were related to the use of medication (Steel et al 1981, Brennan et al 1991). Some antitumor drugs have been shown to cause new cancers (Kaldor et al 1990a,b). L-dopa is responsible, according to one study, for 37% of the original symptoms of elderly people treated for Parkinsonism. Cushing's syndrome is produced by corticosteroids, collagen vascular disease is produced by blood-pressure medications, some cancers have been linked to cholesterol-lowering medicines; the list goes on and on.

A further problem is 'polypharmacy', where a patient takes multiple drugs prescribed by multiple doctors, not all of whom know about each other's prescriptions, or even participation in the treatment of the patient; the results of such unmonitored drug interactions can be, in extreme cases, fatal. Another problem results from the overuse of antibiotics – the development of resistant strains of bacteria. These new strains cause most of the hospital-acquired infections in the US today (Schimmel 1964) and have frightening implications in the field of epidemiology (Garrett 1995). Efforts to deal with drug side-effects have, as the dean of a major school of pharmacy put it, 'fallen flat on their face'.

Non-drug treatments often have side-effects too. Even flawlessly executed major surgery tends to weaken patients' resistance and predispose them to further illness. Radiation exposure in cancer treatment and even in diagnosis has risks as well, and invasive diagnostic procedures like hemodialysis have their dangers.

For all of the risks of these approaches, their rewards are at times unsatisfying. A coronary bypass may not generally reduce the likelihood of another heart attack; and blood pressure goes right back up if medication is stopped. Indeed, another problem of medicine, and in particular of medication, is that it tends to treat symptoms rather than the root causes of disease. When clinical practice consists largely of writing prescriptions for symptoms, it is easy for a physician to begin to feel like a 'pill-pusher'.

Another challenge is functional diseases, such as irritable bowel syndrome and poor digestion. 'Functional', of course, means that we don't see the symptom as a disease; it is considered a normal, if uncomfortable, part of how the body functions. What that might also mean, however, is that Western medicine lacks well-developed theories or methods for treating these ailments. If a patient has a bleeding ulcer, we are trained in what to do; but if the patient merely feels bloated after eating, we may do nothing but tell him that he has no real problem. Yet functional complaints account for one-third of patient visits to family practitioners. This means that, as a practitioner, you must tell a third of your patients either that their problem is psychosomatic ('it's all in your head') or that it is functional (not a real disease) – mainly because medicine doesn't really know how to deal with these problems. Yet it may actually represent a disease, or the precursor of one. Serious diseases do not develop overnight. The lesion that the CAT-scan reveals or the arrhythmia that the EKG measures might have started to develop 10 years before the equipment could have registered any abnormality. During that decade, discomfort may have been dismissed as 'all in your head'. The objective scientific approach to diagnosis may sometimes, ironically, make early detection more difficult.

Finally – and perhaps most importantly – there is the problem of preventive medicine. Aproximately 70% of illnesses are understood to be preventable (National Center for Health Statistics 1992, DHHS 1991, McGinnis 1992); nearly 1 million deaths in the USA every year result from preventable disease (Fries et al 1993). While modern medicine has much to offer here, on the whole its attempts to give guidance in this area remain tentative. Its approach has been piecemeal, based on studying the effects of single substances or factors in isolation (smoking, exercise, cholesterol, saturated fat, and so on) with little sense of an overall ecology of health into which they fit. As a result, for all the useful advances made in recent years, advice on prevention is sometimes contradictory and can be unnervingly volatile. Within the last few years, for example, medical science has been forced to discount claims once made for the beneficial effects of a 30% fat diet, certain vitamin supplements, margarine,

and other purported health factors, and to modify the advice given regarding exercise. And even when we have well-supported advice to give, getting patients to comply is especially challenging.

These are by no means all of the shortcomings that a medical practitioner must deal with. Still, most of us come to agree with Dr Schwarz that we should accept this as just 'reality'. But should we? Or can medicine make significant gains through radically rethinking its approach, or looking into unexpected sources?

We have come to think so. As we will see, MAV addresses all the above issues. It focuses on the root cause of the disease rather than just the symptoms. It reduces dependence on drug therapies and the danger of side-effects. Because it judges every treatment in terms of its effect on the entire mind/body system (see Chapter 5), it reduces the danger of treatment making patients sick. Its potential contribution to preventive medicine is enormous, providing us not only with many new modalities, but with a holistic approach to prevention into which all the parts fit. It can greatly reduce the need to classify a disease as 'functional' with the theory of the three *doshas* and the seven *dhatus* (Ch. 5), and with the subtle diagnostic procedures of MAV (Ch. 6), even subtle disease states can be identified and treated effectively before they develop into more serious problems. This also allows the patient an understanding of his or her symptoms and the underlying imbalance that is causing the symptoms.

The problems of medicine do not reflect on its practitioners, who are idealistic and intelligent; nor are the problems simply a matter of incomplete knowledge, although Western medical knowledge is far less complete than we like to think (the editor of the *British Medical Journal* (Smith 1991) calculated that only 15% of Western medical treatments have a scientific basis or have been definitively demonstrated to be effective). Rather, many of these problems reflect medicine's basic *approach*, its model of health and disease. MAV offers an alternative, fundamentally different approach, and it is this above all that addresses the limitations of the Western medical model.

What do we mean by problems in the basic approach to medicine? For one thing, Western medicine focuses not on health but on disease. During our medical training, the concept of 'health' as a positive entity was not, as far as we can recall, ever treated as a topic. Instead, we, like all medical students, memorized the symptoms of hundreds of diseases. What was health? The absence of these diseases. This is one reason why effective prevention is so hard for modern medicine: if we focus on disease, how can we know how to produce health? It is like trying to get rich by studying poverty.

By contrast, MAV's model begins with an ambitious, detailed concept of what normal health is. The task of the physician begins with seeing how far even a relatively healthy patient has fallen away from that ideal and then doing what is necessary to get him or her back to that state. This is how disease is prevented. This is what allows for an integrated model of preventive medicine. Even in treating disease, the approach emphasizes bringing the patient to a well-defined, well-understood state of healthy balance, in addition to attending to the specific illness.

Another, deeper conceptual problem is that the Western medical approach looks upon the body as a Newtonian machine, whose broken parts can be fixed in isolation. This view is no longer entirely tenable, as Chapter 2 shows, and it stands behind many of the problems of side-effects and iatrogenic illness. Side-effects inevitably result when we treat the body as a machine-like collection of replaceable parts, because the body is not a machine: it is an ecosystem. A drug affects not only the target site, but also everything else; sometimes those other parts are affected negatively. To get beyond side-effects, we need to treat the body as an intelligent, self-interacting system, in which each part affects all other parts. A view that sees that body as a dynamic pattern would be closer to the mark.

HOW A CLINICIAN MIGHT USE MAV: A SCENARIO

To gain more of a sense of what MAV is about, consider the following clinical scenario – involving a disease that is not at all uncommon.

The diagnostic test results leave no doubt: the patient you are treating has hypertension. The standard medical treatment, although it may also recommend that the patient lose weight or use some stress reduction methods, is to control this potentially dangerous condition with medication. Medication, however, has its own dangers as well as compliance problems. The patient may have to try many different anti-hypertensive drugs to minimize such common side-effects as fatigue, impotence, and depression. And even the least troublesome drug has its problems. The hypertension can sometimes become resistant (refractory) to the drug. Patients often become medication-dependent. The treatment does not, in short, treat the causes of the illness, which in this disease can be manifold; it controls the symptom alone.

Suppose, however, that you had been trained in MAV. After the routine Western workup, you would try to address not only the symptoms, but their root causes. You might begin by assessing the state of balance of subtle homeostatic aspects of the patient's mind/body (Ch. 5). To do this, you would use non-invasive diagnostic techniques that greatly extend Western diagnostics (Ch. 6). Hypertension can have many causes, but the root cause always involves some subtle inner imbalance; treating that can always help, and can often solve the problem.

Once you have identified the nature of the imbalances, you have a range of natural modalities available for restoring the patient's normal inner balance. You can recommend some surprisingly effective changes in diet (Ch. 7), daily routine (Ch. 9), and exercise (Ch. 11). You can recommend herbal supplements, which some medical research has shown to have remarkable effects, which include alleviating cancer conditions, and also reducing cardiovascular risk factors (Ch. 8). Some of these affect homeostatic mechanisms that govern blood pressure. You would recommend Transcendental Meditation (see Ch. 3), which research has shown to be unusually effective in reducing hypertension and other cardiovascular risk factors (Schneider et al 1992, 1995). And you would likely recommend *panchakarma*, a detoxifying therapy that can also be very useful in treating high blood pressure, and which has been shown to reduce other cardiovascular risk factors (Ch. 10; Sharma et al 1993). And you would have a wide range of other MAV modalities available as well: aroma therapies, music therapies, exercise programs using neuromuscular and neurorespiratory integration exercises, and more.

For the patient, the results can be vastly more satisfactory than a lifetime of medication dependence and side-effects. The root cause of the hypertension can be removed, not only without side-effects, but with side benefits, such as improved energy and sense of well-being, and reduced likelihood of other disease.

MAHARISHI'S VEDIC APPROACH TO HEALTH

In the last few years, Maharishi has placed MAV into a larger context, Maharishi's Vedic Approach to Health. The Vedic Approach to Health includes all of what is in this book, but much else as well; we discuss some of its additional elements in the final chapter. The Vedic Approach emphasizes above all, though, that the basis of health is consciousness. According to Maharishi, 'There is an inseparable, very intimate relationship between the unmanifest field of consciousness and all the manifest levels of the physiology: that is why Maharishi's Vedic Approach to Health handles the field of health primarily from the most basic area of health – the field of consciousness – through the natural approach of consciousness, Transcendental Meditation' (Maharishi Mahesh Yogi 1995).

Maharishi continues by noting that his Vedic Approach also handles health from the more expressed levels of health, the physiology, behavior and environment; from the field of knowledge; and even from the relationship of the individual to the cosmos. But the previous quote must intrigue some readers. What exactly is meant by the *unmanifest* field of consciousness? What sort of relationship could it have to the body? We will explore that in our next two chapters.

REFERENCES

Bates D W, Cullen D J, Laird N et al 1995 Incidence of adverse drug events and potential adverse drug events. Journal of the American Medical Association 274(1):29–34

Brennan T A, Leape L L, Laird N M et al 1991 Incidence of adverse events and negligence in hospitalized patients. New England Journal of Medicine 324(6):370–376

DHHS 1991 Healthy people 2000. Government Printing Office, Washington DC

Friend T 1995 Using drugs 'off label'. Doctors 'doing things they can't back up'. USA Today, 12 September, pp 1A–2A

Fries J F, Koop C E, Beadle C E et al, 1993 Reducing health care costs by reducing the need and demand for medical services. New England Journal of Medicine 329(5):321–325

Garrett L 1995 The coming plague. Basic Books, New York

Isselbacher K J, Braunwald E, Wilson J D, Martin J B, Fauci A S, Kasper D L (eds) 1994 Harrison's principles of internal medicine, 13th edn. McGraw-Hill, New York, p 405

Johnson J A, Bootman J L 1995 Drug-related morbidity and mortality. Archives of Internal Medicine 155:1949–1956

Kaldor J M, Day N E, Clarke E A et al 1990a Leukemia following Hodgkin's disease. New England Journal of Medicine 322(1):7–13

Kaldor J M, Day N E, Pettersson F et al 1990b Leukemia following chemotherapy for ovarian cancer. New England Journal of Medicine 322(1):1–6

Leape L L 1994 Error in medicine. Journal of the American Medical Association 272(23):1851–1857

McGinnis J M 1992 Investing in health: the role of disease prevention. In: Bland R H, Bonnicksen A L (eds) Emerging issues in biomedical policy, vol 1. Columbia University Press, New York, pp 13–26

Maharishi Mahesh Yogi 1995 Maharishi's Vedic Approach to Health. Maharishi Vedic University Press Vlodrop, Netherlands, p.10

National Center for Health Statistics 1992 Health United States, 1991. Hyattsville Md (Public Health Service DHHS publication no. (PHS) 92–1232)

Robin E D 1987 Iatroepidemics: a probe to examine systematic preventable errors in (chest) medicine. American Review of Respiratory Disease 135(5):1152–1156

Schimmel E M 1964 The hazards of hospitalization. Annals of Internal Medicine 60(1):100–110

Schneider, R H, Alexander C N, Wallace R K 1992 In search of an optimal behavioral treatment for hypertension: a review and focus on Transcendental Meditation. In: Johnson E H, Gentry W D, Julius S (eds) Personality, elevated blood pressure, and essential hypertension. Hemisphere, Washington DC, pp 123–131

Schneider R H Staggers F, Alexander C N et al 1995 Stress reduction for the treatment of hypertension in elderly African-Americans: a randomized, controlled trial of Transcendental Meditation and Progressive Muscle Relaxation. Hypertension 26(5):820–827

Sharma H M, Nidich S I, Sands D, Smith D E 1993 Improvement in cardiovascular risk factors through Panchakarma purification procedures. Journal of Research and Education in Indian Medicine 12(4):3–13

Smith R 1991 Where is the wisdom? The poverty of medical evidence. British Medical Journal 303:798–799

Steel K, Gertman P M, Crescenzi C, Anderson J 1981 Iatrogenic illness on a general medical service at a university hospital. New England Journal of Medicine 304(11):638–642

2

The 'consciousness model' of medicine

Classical Ayurvedic texts say that to treat a patient with complete effectiveness, you must treat the patient not as a set of parts, but as a whole. How do they characterize that wholeness? Each of us has, the texts say, three aspects: consciousness, mind, and body; and truly complete medical care must address all three of them.

Attention to that first dimension is what distinguishes Maharishi Ayur-Veda (MAV). MAV makes consciousness its central focus. By no means does it neglect the other two dimensions, mind and body, and much of this book describes its theories and treatment modalities for them. But the body, it says, is the tip of the iceberg, and the mind only a slightly submerged part of it; the major part is consciousness. MAV sees consciousness as the very foundation of the patient and, therefore, of medical treatment.

What is meant here by 'consciousness'? Nowadays, the term is used to refer to all sorts of things: a political attitude, perhaps, or an information processing mode, or recognition of some fact of life. In MAV it refers to something much more basic. Consciousness is that which is most intimate to our experience – that which lies beneath thought and feeling. It is *awareness* itself, the experiencer. If you had to give up one of your mental faculties, it is the last thing you would sacrifice, for without awareness nothing else would register.

Awareness is so intimate to us that we take it for granted. Philosophers, however, have puzzled over it for centuries, and some today recognize that it is one of the ultimate mysteries of fundamental science (Searle 1995, Chalmers 1995). MAV says that there is much more to it than most of us have experienced, or than science has yet uncovered – though, as this book shows, some of the most advanced areas of science are beginning to come to a similar outlook.

Regarding consciousness, MAV states first that our ordinary experience of consciousness is at best a glimpse of what is possible; it is, indeed, substandard. In ordinary experience, the Self – the underlying experiencer, the silent witness – is hidden. We experience thoughts, feelings, sensations, and perceptions, but not the experiencer. This is so familiar a state of affairs that it may seem not worth mentioning outside of a philosophy classroom; but to MAV it is profoundly significant. The hiding of one's essential inner nature is, as we will see, considered to be the ultimate basis of disease and problems in life.

Second, this silent witness – the quiet, simplest state of awareness that is usually hidden, even though it is centrally there in our lives – has, according to MAV, a profound status. It is our deepest connection to the universe, to all the laws of nature. Its implications go far beyond our own mental experience to include the totality of life.

A book on Maharishi Ayur-Veda must begin by explaining these points.

PURE CONSCIOUSNESS AS THE UNIFIED FIELD

The Vedic tradition understands that nature is not fundamentally objective. It is not based on material objects. Rather, the most fundamental reality is said to be completely subjective – an unbounded and eternal field of pure, abstract intelligence, or consciousness. This unified field is the home of all the laws of nature. What we see as the material world is, in reality, waves, or fluctuations, or impulses, of this non-material, underlying field of pure consciousness. What we ourselves are – or more exactly, what our minds and bodies are – is pure intelligence in motion.

In the Vedic understanding, if the human mind becomes still and pure enough, it can contact this pure field of consciousness at the basis of the physical world. It can settle down to become directly aware of it.

Having this experience may seem like an interesting possibility, but MAV goes much further. It considers this experience necessary for creating ideal health. In Vedic thought, the benefits of direct experience of the

unified field are held to be so great that they are said to give rise to distinctly higher states of consciousness, collectively called 'enlightenment'.

The Vedic tradition has a terminology for these phenomena. The simplest form of our own awareness – pure consciousness – is called our *atman* (or 'Self'). Vedic thought expresses the *atman's* status in the expression *Ayam Ātmā Brahm*: this *atman* is *Brahman* ('totality', the unified field). The process of growing to the state known as 'enlightenment' involves the *atman* (the Self of everyone) awakening to its full status as *Brahman* (the Self of the universe).

Enlightenment

In the Vedic usage, 'enlightenment' does not refer to the possession of facts, or of a belief system, or of any other intellectual understanding whatsoever. Rather, it refers to 'light' from within. It means the individual mind is fully illuminated by the transcendental, infinite field of pure consciousness at the basis of nature.

Like a tree reaching its roots down to an underground reservoir, the human mind can, as we said, settle down to experience this infinite field of pure intelligence. Maharishi explains that, by repeating this experience twice daily with the Transcendental Meditation and TM-Sidhi program, the mind gains familiarity with this field. It gains the ability to maintain contact with the unified field even while going about its daily business. Says Maharishi:

It's only in the beginning days of meditation that one has to meditate in order to experience that silent, quiet level of the mind, that state of pure consciousness. As we continue to alternate the experience of meditation with daily activity, the value of that pure consciousness is infused into the mind. The pure level of consciousness becomes stabilized in our awareness. And when that pure level . . . is a living reality even during daily activity, this is the state of enlightenment. This is life free from suffering, life when every thought and action is spontaneously correct. (Quoted in Oates 1986, pp 33–34).

Among other things, the state of enlightenment is regarded as the optimum state of human health. Thus bringing it about is the highest goal of MAV. Why would enlightenment, or even growing towards it, benefit health? There are several reasons, which we will look at one by one.

ACTION IN ACCORD WITH NATURAL LAW

The last remark in the Maharishi quote – about 'spontaneously correct' thought and action – should be discussed further. A statement from the Ṛk Veda (1.158.6) expresses it as *Yatīnāṁ Brahmā bhavati sārathiḥ*; Maharishi's translation is: 'For those whose minds are established in self-referral consciousness, the infinite organizing power of natural law becomes the charioteer.' In this state of life, daily living is said to be guided spontaneously by the laws of nature.

One might object that all actions are in accordance with the laws of physics, biology, etc.; but Vedic science uses the terms in another sense. Some actions produce desirable, life-supporting outcomes by taking all such laws into account, and some produce undesirable outcomes by not considering the consequences of the laws of nature. If one walks off the edge of a roof, one's fall is governed by the law of gravity, but one has acted 'out of accordance' with its consequences. If one takes care to avoid falling off roofs, one is acting 'in accordance' with gravity's consequences. Certain laws of nature imply actions that uphold well-being and evolution – e.g. caring for one's children – and also opposite actions that would cause unhappiness and harm. Acting spontaneously in accordance with natural law means spontaneously acting in a way that supports well-being.

This accordance with natural law also is said to have a dynamic effect in daily, moment-to-moment activity. Great athletes often describe an experience of going 'into the zone', where, for a few moments, every action is automatic and spontaneously right. This is a taste of enlightenment – an idea of what is meant by 'life lived spontaneously in full accord with the laws of nature'. When the mind is in tune with pure consciousness – the unified field of natural law – then thought and action are computed and supported by all the laws of nature.

This phenomenon of spontaneous right action has an important implication for health. Maintaining health results from living in accordance with the laws of nature that govern the operation of the human body. The human body is not designed, for example, to inhale tobacco smoke, so when it is subjected to that unnatural activity, the lungs and heart are damaged.

Acting in accordance with natural law here [...] smoking. As this suggests, many of these [...] nature governing health can be identified: d[...] smoke, get some exercise, etc. But, inevitably, a grea[t] many laws can't. Medical science knows, at this point, only so much; MAV gives a good deal of additional advice (covered in later chapters). But all its advice must be suited to the situation and the individual, and, besides, many more issues will arise that no one has foreseen. The ideal solution would be to be able to act spontaneously in accordance with natural law. MAV holds that one can gain that spontaneous ability by developing one's inner awareness, one's direct experience of the state of transcendental consciousness. This 'awakening' of one's consciousness to its full status as the unified field is said to produce a spontaneous, intuitive alignment with natural law. (This may account for the finding that TM is helpful in quitting smoking, overcoming drug and alcohol dependencies, and in general improving compliance rates in preventive medicine: for a review, see Alexander et al 1994.)

FROM CONSCIOUSNESS TO MIND TO BODY: A MORE DETAILED VIEW OF THE CONSCIOUSNESS MODEL OF MAV

To explain the idea that enlightenment brings spontaneous attunement to natural law, as defined above, we need to go in more detail into Vedic Science.

The idea that reconnecting to the simplest form of awareness, pure consciousness, will bring a deeper attunement to the flow of evolution in nature depends on the idea that it is the unified field that gives rise to nature in the first place. Connecting to consciousness is like plugging in to the central processing unit of the laws of nature. Maharishi's Vedic Science explains it as follows.

VEDA AND PHYSICS

First, a slight detour. Unfamiliar though the Vedic worldview may sound to Western ears, it is remarkably congruent with the view of nature that physics has uncovered. Physics too describes the apparently d us as in reality just the … underlying non-material

… direction involved what is … Quantum mechanics found … are really 'wave functions' on underlying … ds. Unlike classical particles, the wave functions are not what we usually think of as 'things'. They are, essentially, *knowledge* – they represent the *probability* that something will occur. When you think that the world is made of probability functions, the universe begins to seem not like a giant machine, as it seemed in Newtonian physics, but like an idea – in fact, like expressed knowledge. The physicist Henry P. Stapp of Lawrence Berkeley Laboratory says:

In view of these uniformly idea-like characteristics of the quantum-physical world, the proper answer to our question, 'What sort of world do we live in?' would seem to be this: 'We live in an idea-like world, not a matter-like world'...There is, in fact, in the quantum universe no natural place for matter. This conclusion, curiously, is the exact reverse of the circumstance that in the classical physical universe there was not a natural place for mind. (Stapp 1993, p. 211)

The next step in physical understanding was seeing that the various quantum fields arise from a smaller number of underlying fields. In the 1960s, physicists showed that electromagnetism and 'weak' interactions, two of the four basic 'force' fields, were really just one field in different guises. Similarly, the myriad elementary parti-cles (neutrinos, quarks and so on) have now been shown to all be fluctuations of one 'matter' field, which is called the 'lepto-quark' field (Fig. 2.1). In fact, physics now sees all the forces and particles of nature as fluctuations of three 'superfields'. (We will look at the superfields in more detail in a later chapter, as they turn out to have striking parallels to MAV concepts.)

The leading quest in physics today is to find, lying beneath the three superfields, one single 'superunified' field. Many physicists believe they have the gist of a successful unified field theory, which is called 'superstring theory'. Some feel that they should have its details worked out within a decade (Mukerjee 1996). If so, physics will be describing everything in nature, including our bodies, as the modes of vibration of an underlying, transcendental, non-material unity – modes of vibration on an underlying field of pure intelligence.

Vedic thought can be seen to have always described the universe in these terms. Many parallels have been drawn between the Vedic description of the unified field and the emerging one in physics (Hagelin 1987). These often involve the mechanics of how unity manifests itself into diversity in the first place. We will look first at the Vedic Science approach and then explore its parallels in physics.

The mechanics of creation

How is it that a unity at the basis of nature, an

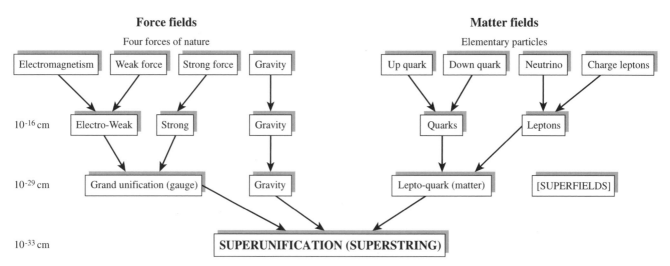

Figure 2.1 Unification of the fundamental force and matter fields in the unified field

unchanging field of pure potential, would manifest into diversity? The Vedic Science explanation is as follows. The very nature of the unified field as pure consciousness must mean, of course, that it is *conscious*. It is aware. And if, at the basis of creation, consciousness is the sole reality, then it has only itself to be aware of. Because of its own nature, Maharishi maintains that pure consciousness 'cannot hold itself back' from knowing itself; it is, therefore, 'completely self-referral' – aware of itself alone. Thus the very nature of consciousness ensures that an undifferentiated unity – pure consciousness – automatically becomes a tripartite diversity. As consciousness knows itself, it becomes knower, process of knowing, and known – or observer, process of observation, and observed. Consciousness is the subject, object, and connection between the two. It is both one and three at the same time.

In Sanskrit, the knower is termed *rishi*, the process of knowing, *devata*, and the object of knowledge *chhandas*. The underlying unity from which the three arise (and in which they continue to exist) is termed *samhita* (unitedness, collectedness).

There is a further step in the process. In the field of pure consciousness, Maharishi states, the oneness or *samhita* and the three, *rishi*, *devata* and *chhandas* (the knower, process of knowing, and known) – all three of which are really just different shades of the *samhita* – alternate back and forth with what is called 'infinite frequency' (Fig. 2.2). This rapid alternation between the unity and its trinity imparts an infinite dynamism to a field otherwise absolutely silent. In Maharishi's understanding, this is where the variety of creation begins. The unity or singularity of pure consciousness spontaneously 'breaks' into diversity, the silence of pure consciousness into dynamism.

From consciousness to matter

Not only is the 'symmetry breaking' of the unified field a spontaneous process, it is also sequential. Once this internal self-referral process of elaboration begins, it continues indefinitely, creating the complexity of the universe. The sequentially elaborating interactions between *rishi*, *devata*, and *chhandas* are, says Maharishi, 'those fine creative impulses that are engaged in transforming the field of intelligence into the field of matter'.

To explore this last point, the early steps of the sequence of elaboration generate what becomes mental reality: I-ness (*ahamkara* or ego), and then intellect (*buddhi*), the faculty that discriminates. It is *buddhi* that stands at the junction point of unity and diversity, one and three, *samhita* and *rishi*, *devata*, and *chhandas*.

Eventually, after a number of intermediate steps, the sequential unfoldment gives rise to matter (Fig. 2.3). Matter first precipitates in the form of five *mahabhutas*; these are examined in Chapter 5, where we see that they are strikingly parallel to the five 'spin types' of physics. From the five *mahabhutas*, a further elabora-

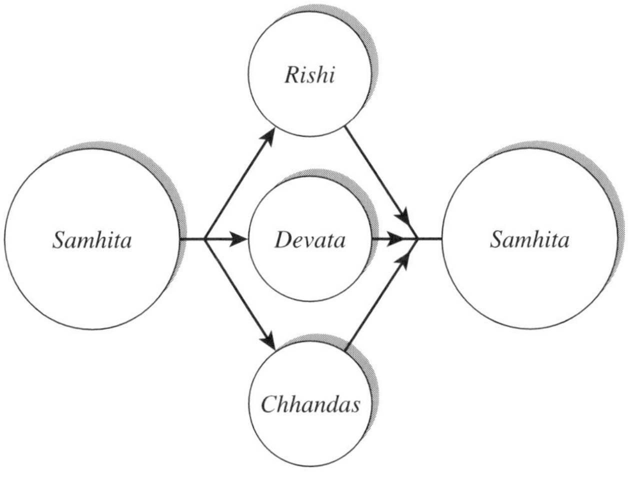

Figure 2.2 The alternation between *samhita* and *rishi*, *devata*, and *chhandas*

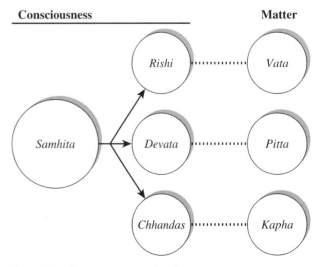

Figure 2.3 Consciousness and matter

tion leads to their combinations into three physical principles called the three *doshas* (which are explained in detail in Chapter 5, and parallel the three superfields). The *doshas* are the governing principles of the body. Again, there are many other steps in this sequential elaboration, but for the purposes of this book, the above will suffice.

This discussion brings us back to the tripod that we began this chapter with – the three dimensions that an MAV physician must deal with: consciousness, mind, and body. Why must we deal with all three? The reason is that consciousness is ultimately the source of the mind *and* of the body. The body is a precipitate of the subjective realm (here we have one key element of why thoughts and feelings can have such a potent influence on the physiology). The mind manifests before body, and the body manifests from it.

We compared the unified field to an underground reservoir from which the tree can draw sustenance; the faculties of the mind might, in this analogy, be compared to the roots. Clearly, these roots can affect the tree significantly. Awakening the mind to its full unbounded status by re-enlivening its connection to the unified field nourishes health from its most basic level. This is why MAV places so much emphasis on the Transcendental Meditation and TM-Sidhi programs, which we discuss in our next chapter.

How manifestation occurs: physics and Vedic Science compared

Does this have any correspondences in the physics of the unified field? To review: in Vedic Science, the unified field manifests as follows:

1. 'Symmetry breaking': trifurcation, caused by the nature of the unified field as consciousness, into a state of one (*samhita*) and three (knower, process of knowing, and known, or *rishi*, *devata*, and *chhandas*) at the same time.
2. These three values interact with each other to generate new generations of *rishi*, *devata*, and *chhandas*.
3. This interaction of *rishi*, *devata* and *chhandas* is a sequential process of elaboration which finally results in the emergence of matter.

As it happens, like Vedic Science, physics describes the superunified field as having a 'three in one' nature; as being both infinitely silent and infinitely dynamic; and as manifesting through a process of 'spontaneous sequential symmetry breaking' (Hagelin 1987). We will not go into the mathematical details of the physics, but the parallels are striking.

VEDA AND PHYSIOLOGY

Physics describes the world as the modes of vibration of a single, transcendental unified field of pure knowledge. This is almost the exact wording of the Vedic description. Indeed, it is implicit in the word 'Veda' itself. We might assume that the Vedas are simply a collection of ancient books. In fact, though, the word *Veda* means 'knowledge', and, according to Maharishi, refers to transcendental packets of knowledge that are held, indeed, to be the modes of 'vibration' of the unified field. These 'modes of vibration' of the unified field, the elements of the Veda, are what manifest into the material world around us. The Veda is an abstract blueprint of creation, or, in Maharishi Mahesh Yogi's more dynamic metaphor, the 'constitution' of the universe – the comparison being with the constitution of a government, the basis of national laws (which in this metaphor stand for natural laws).

We might think of the contents of Veda as the laws of nature, expressed not in equations but rather as vibrations (these, according to Vedic Science, can be heard as sounds when one's awareness is sufficiently established in transcendental consciousness). The Ṛk Veda, for example, records the alternations of *rishi*, *devata*, and *chhandas* that are described above. This is why the mind awakening to its full status as the unified field results in life spontaneously in tune with natural law: the mind at this level of dignity contains all the laws of nature within its most silent, settled state.

The idea that the laws of nature structuring the body are vibrant in the unified field is given with some specificity in Vedic Science. The Vedic tradition locates 40 basic types of modes of vibration of the unified field; the first of the 40 is the totality; the other 39 are the structuring dynamics of that holistic value. Then there are divisions and subdivisions of these values. These modes of vibration are expressed in the 40 branches of the Vedic literature, and have been shown to have extraordinarily detailed one-to-one correspondence with 40 aspects of human physiology and anatomy. (All of these correspondences are elaborated in Maharishi's Vedic Approach to Health: see Nader 1995 and Nader, in press.)

This correspondence has an important implication for MAV: it adds a deeper reason why experiencing transcendental consciousness is so important to health.

RESETTING THE SEQUENCE

We talked about the unified field manifesting into creation through 'spontaneous, sequential symmetry breaking'. The *sequential* element is crucial. The fluctuations of the unified field, we said, elaborate in a sequence. Ill health, Vedic Science holds, results from the *disturbance* of the normal sequence in the expression of natural law. A degenerative disease, for example, is ultimately the result of the proper sequence of natural law being disrupted. Restoring health is the result of restoring the proper sequential unfoldment of natural law.

How can the sequence be restored? If all the laws of nature arise from the unified field, and the mind can settle down to its own simplest state of awareness, transcendental consciousness, and realize that it is the unified field, then, in this state, it is one with the home of all the laws of nature. These include the laws of nature that give rise to the body. The way to reset the correct sequence of expression of natural law, the sequence that creates a healthy body, is to restore one's connection to the unified field from which the laws of nature arise – that is, to experience transcendental consciousness.

Subjectively, transcendental consciousness is a state of 'pure consciousness' – consciousness aware of itself alone, awake to its own unbounded nature; it is a state, also, as Vedic texts put it, of *ananda*, bliss or pure happiness. Objectively, however, this subjective state correlates with a remarkably orderly and settled state of the physiology, which has been both identified scientifically and associated with significant benefits to health (this is explored in detail in Chapter 3). In both respects, subjective and objective, the experience promotes healing and health.

In addition to Transcendental Meditation and other mental techniques, other elements of MAV, such as diet, herbs, and primordial sound therapy, all of which we will discuss in later chapters, are used to restore the proper sequence.

This idea of resetting the sequence is also what explains the spontaneous attunement with natural law that results from transcendental consciousness becoming established in the awareness. As the laws of nature evolve the universe in a sequence, the individual gains the full support of the proper sequence of laws of nature. The athlete's timing becomes perfect, as he or she correctly calculates the exact force and angle for each shot and each step. And the patient correctly calculates the behaviour necessary for health.

PRAGYA-APARADH: HOW WE 'FORGET' THE UNIFIED FIELD

We have reviewed the reasons why Vedic Science considers growing to enlightenment by awakening the individual mind and Self to their full status as the unified field (*Brahman* or 'totality') to be the basis of perfect health. Doing so leads one to act spontaneously in accordance with natural law; and it restores the expression of the proper sequence of natural law that gives rise to perfect health. The body is considered to be, in these specific ways, an expression of the unified field. Enlivening our conscious connection to that field is thus said to have a healing and health-promoting influence on the body. It enlivens the order, the patterns, that should prevail in a healthy body – the body being thought of as, essentially, not matter so much as sequentially unfolded patterns of intelligence.

But how could the sequence be disrupted in the first place – or, to put it differently, how do we lose our 'memory' of our status as the unified field?

Maharishi begins his analysis of this with a key aspect of the interaction of the threefold nature of the unified field that we discussed earlier: *rishi*, *devata* and *chhandas*. He calls these three entities 'intellectually conceived components' of the unified field of consciousness. By saying that the observer, the process of observation, and the observed are 'intellectually conceived components', Maharishi is emphasizing that they are products of intellectual discrimination, rather than phenomena with absolute existence. By 'intellect' – *buddhi* – is meant something deeper than the faculty measured on IQ tests; rather, it refers to the faculty that draws distinctions and discriminates. It stands, as we said, at the junction of *samhita* (unity) with *rishi*, *devata*, and *chhandas* (diversity).

In Maharishi's explanation, manifestation into the material universe creates no difficulty as long as the intellect does not get lost in its own discriminations. But as a sandstorm can hide the landscape, the swirl of dynamic interactions among *rishi*, *devata*, and *chhandas* can hide the ultimate reality. The intellect gets lost in the complex, ever-changing vision of the world. Consciousness becomes object-referral instead of self-referral, lost in the masking value of *chhandas* (the object of knowing). The glamour of the material creation fills the mind. The memory of the silent unity of consciousness – the *samhita* of *rishi*, *devata*, and *chhandas* – disappears. This one-sided awareness is called *pragya-aparadh*, the 'mistake of the intellect' (Fig. 2.4).

The problem, again, is not the diversification, the manifestation of pure consciousness into matter; rather it is the forgetting of the underlying unity, while enjoying the material expressions, that constitutes the 'mistake'. Our enjoyment and engagement with diversity is no problem in itself, but becomes one when the unity is forgotten. This 'loss of memory', as it is called in Vedic Science, leads to faulty judgment of how to act with regards to health and other areas of life (i.e. to act out of accordance with natural law): one makes one's choices only in terms of the five senses, rather than in terms of the totality of life. One might, for example, choose to eat too much unhealthy food, or to work too hard and neglect one's sleep, or in some other way to indulge in behavior that contributes to disease. It also leads to the loss of the correct sequential expression of natural law in the body.

Thus, according to MAV, *pragya-aparadh* is the basis of the etiology of all disease: it both predisposes one to lifestyle choices that undermine health, and undermines the expression of natural intelligence in the body. When *pragya-aparadh* is reversed, by contrast, it is the basis of all cure, and indeed of vastly improved life in many respects. The technologies of consciousness of MAV, the subject of our next chapter, are designed to overcome *pragya-aparadh* – to 'restore memory' of the unified field.

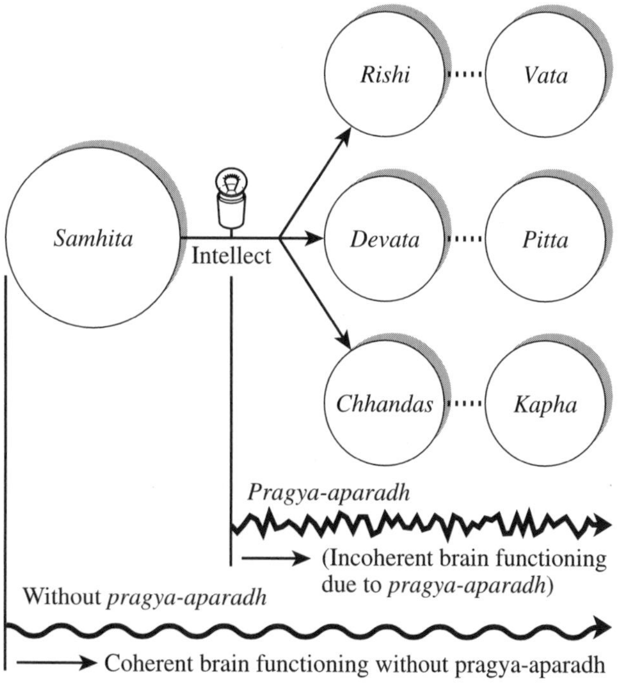

THE IMPLICATIONS FOR MEDICINE: THE BODY AS STANDING WAVES

Pragya-aparadh, the mistake of the intellect, is an essentially universal situation today. Aside from the resulting ill health, it has a more abstract implication: that our normal, commonsense view of the world is mistaken. The world we normally see is a grand illusion (the Vedic term for this is *maya*). The apparently solid objects around us are not solid at all, but waves on a non-material field. The diversity of the surface around us arises from a hidden, underlying unity.

The view physics is arriving at of this underlying unity accords in outline, and even in detail, with the Vedic view of reality. Realizing that the apparently solid objects around us are nothing but fluctuations in the non-material unified field, physicists have understood that material creation is an illusion created by our senses and our interpretations. This has been discussed at length by Sir James Jeans, Sir Arthur Eddington, Werner Heisenberg, Erwin Schrödinger, and many other prominent 20th-century physicists. None, however, has stated the conclusion more firmly

Figure 2.4 *Pragya-aparadh*: the source of all disorder and disease

than Paul Davies: the 'commonsense world of experience is a sham' (Davies 1985, p 37).

Modern medical science, however, continues to subscribe to the classical way of thinking, which accords with the commonsense world of experience. Medicine thinks of the body as a complex machine. The body is made of solid matter; it can get out of tune; it can be attacked by outside agents. To fix it when it is 'broken', you shoot magic bullets (drugs) at the attackers, or cut and paste the machine together as if it were an auto engine in need of better wiring or a new piston.

For much of what medicine does, such a view seems to suffice. But as we saw in Chapter 1, the view has its limits. The ubiquitous problem of side-effects, and some of the problems of iatrogenic illness, can be said to result from seeing the body in terms of a machine made of independent parts rather than as a holistic pattern.

After all, the descriptions from quantum physics and from MAV paint quite a different picture. This suggests a very different way of understanding the body. The body is not a machine. It is an immensely complex flux of vibrations in an underlying non-material unified field of pure intelligence. Classical physics thinks of molecules as small agglomerations of solid matter, like billiard balls held together by magnetic attraction. But in the more accurate quantum view, a molecule is not a collection of billiard balls, but a *pattern* of fluctuation in this underlying non-material field.

Think of it this way. If you drive a pole into the bed of a stream, standing it up straight, the water washing by it will create a 'standing wave' on the downstream side of the pole. Water that has separated to move around the pole rushes together again, creating a crest. This standing wave appears to have a constant shape and a continuous existence, but in fact the water flowing through is new every instant.

Molecules can be thought of as standing waves.

They appear solid and unchanging, but in fact, they are simply fluctuations of the underlying quantum field. The individual atoms and particles come and go, replacing one another continually; only the underlying pattern remains the same. The same is true of the body as a whole. Some atoms are replaced every few days or even every few minutes. In this flux of constant change all that remains the same is the immensely complex standing wave. The body is a pattern, not a hunk of material.

This implies, among other things, that health care should change drastically. Superficial approaches will still have utility: if you break your leg, you'll still need a cast. At macroscopic time and distance scales, the kind we're used to dealing with, the 'classical' picture of a billiard-ball world is approximately correct. But as we discuss in Chapter 8, a major advance in medicine, the understanding of 'free radicals', has come from looking past the cellular level and to the level of molecules. This raises the question of whether equally great advances could come from looking even deeper, to the field on which molecules – which are really just 'standing waves' – have their basis.

This implies that a fully effective health-care system would not function only at the gross material level. Instead, it would also function at the most basic level of the laws of nature. It would function from both the surface and the depths. The aim of MAV is to supply such an integrated approach. The main concern of the MAV model is, as outlined above, consciousness and how it relates to health. One might even call the MAV model 'the consciousness model' of medicine. The following chapters will explore its many avenues. The first, and most basic, is the method that operates on the most basic level, that of consciousness itself: Transcendental Meditation. Does this offer any evidence for this 'consciousness' paradigm, or for 'higher states of consciousness'? These questions are examined in the next chapter.

REFERENCES

Alexander C N, Robinson P, Rainforth M 1994 Treating and preventing alcohol, nicotine and drug abuse through Transcendental Meditation: a review and statistical meta-analysis. Alcoholism Treatment Quarterly 11 (1/2):13–87
Chalmers, D J 1995 The puzzle of conscious experience. Scientific American 273(6):80–86

Davies P 1985 Superforce: the search for a grand unified theory of nature. Touchstone, Simon & Schuster, New York
Davies P 1992 The matter myth: dramatic discoveries that challenge our understanding of physical reality. Simon & Schuster, New York
Hagelin J S 1987 Is consciousness the unified field? A field theorist's perspective. Modern Science and Vedic Science 1: 29–87

Mukerjee M 1996 'Explaining everything.' Scientific American 274 (1):88–94

Nader T 1995 Human physiology: expression of Veda and the Vedic literature. Maharishi Vedic University, Vlodrop, Netherlands

Nader T (in press) Human physiology: expression of Veda and the Vedic literature, revised edn. Maharishi Vedic University, Vlodrop, Netherlands

Oates R M Jr 1986 Celebrating the dawn. Putnam, New York.

Searle J 1995 'The Mystery of Consciousness' New York Review of Books, 2 November, pp 60 ff

Stapp H P 1993 Mind, matter and quantum mechanics. Springer-Verlag, Berlin

3

A practical application of the consciousness model: Transcendental Meditation

In the previous chapter, we employed a comparison of the body to 'standing waves' on an underlying field of pure consciousness. This chapter will look at the main technique in Maharishi Ayur-Veda (MAV) for accessing this underlying field, the Transcendental Meditation (TM) technique.

TM was brought to the West in 1958 by Maharishi Mahesh Yogi, whose teaching differed from the teaching that was common at the time. He consistently urged a new understanding of meditation, which at the time was generally considered to be impractical, a way of escaping from the realities of life. MAV posits that the Transcendental Meditation technique is not mystical, and that it is not a religion – it requires no belief, for one thing – but a practical technology to increase success in daily life. Meditation was also, at the time, expected to be difficult, and to take years of effort to master. But correct practice of Transcendental Meditation, involves no concentration or mental effort. It is natural and effortless and easy to learn. Also, it requires only 20 minutes practice twice a day, which is done sitting comfortably.

TM involves the use of mantras – sounds whose vibratory effects on the nervous system are said to be especially beneficial – and here again the MAV approach is different from the usual. In Transcendental Meditation, the mantra is not something one aims to concentrate one's mind upon. The term 'transcendental' indicates that in TM the mind *transcends* even the subtlest impulses of the mantra and other thought.

The idea of mantras can be new to some Westerners so a few additional words of explanation may be useful. One key principle behind mantras is that *sounds have an effect on the physiology*. This principle is used, in

MAV's music therapy and primordial sound therapy (Ch. 13). But both these therapies use *external* sounds. Obviously, externally generated sounds can have either a soothing effect (think of the sounds of a flowing brook) or a jarring one, such as the proverbial fingernail on the chalkboard (in Chapter 13 we also examine scientific research showing how sounds may be able to affect physiology at the molecular level). The mantras used in TM, however, are 'heard' *mentally*, as thoughts or faint ideas, rather than being spoken out or listened to. This is because, again, they are meant as vehicles to allow the mind to transcend conscious thought. Speaking them externally would make the inward settling of the mind more difficult. According to MAV, mentally generated sounds have as much of an effect on the nervous system as externally generated ones – in some ways, a greater effect. A thought, according to the Vedic approach, is a very subtle, semi-manifest object. Thus, a premium is placed on using mantras whose effects on the nervous system are beneficial. During TM, the mind experiences finer and finer states of the mantra until it finally transcends conscious thought. The subtler states of a suitable mantra, and experience of transcendental consciousness, according to Vedic tradition produce a profound healing effect on the physiology.

More than that, mantras have to be suitable for the individual in question. Some mantras, for example, are specifically suited to religious renunciates, and are not considered appropriate for those engaged in activity in the world. Teachers of TM are trained to choose mantras to suit the individual. Their choice is guided by specific criteria derived from the ancient oral tradition of meditation instruction in the Vedic tradition. To learn to teach TM, teachers undergo extensive training. Maharishi began training teachers in the 1960s; TM teacher-training courses currently last approximately 1 year, and are held worldwide. The course involves training in the field of consciousness, both in its theoretical and practical aspects. Only after one has demonstrated success in both areas does one become qualified to teach TM.

Mantra selection is only a small part of the process of TM teacher training. When students start using the mantra a host of new questions arise as a result of new mental and physiological experiences; a TM teacher learns how to deal with these in one-to-one interaction with the student, based on the student's needs. This has been found to be the only way to convey effectively the effortless but subtle technique of allowing the mind to transcend on the mantra. This is why simply printing a list of mantras would be of no value; one could not convey in print the proper technique for using them, so they would be useless. That is why the mantras are kept confidential and are only imparted in the context of learning how to teach the technique of using them. Using the mantra incorrectly will not lead to transcending. (It is often difficult for some to understand the value of oral traditions of imparting knowledge, but this is one example of an area in which oral instruction has crucial advantages.) Some physicians have questioned whether using the 'correct' mantra really matters; the issue has not been subjected yet to a thorough research program, but we will see later that research so far supports the idea that using the correct mantra matters a great deal.

Again, the purpose of mantras is to give the mind a vehicle to transcend not only the mantra, but the entire thinking process. MAV describes the resulting experience of Transcendental Meditation as one of profound inner silence – with the mind wide awake, but perfectly still. In this view, this simplest state of awareness is the source of thought, and is considered to be identical to the unified field. With a correct meditation technique, the human mind will settle down effortlessly to this silent state, motivated by the mind's own natural tendencies.

One other new angle that MAV brought to meditation was to encourage scientists to research it. About a decade after Maharishi arrived in the US, the first study was undertaken. In the late 1960s, Dr R. Keith Wallace, a physiologist working at UCLA, did a series of experiments, which were published from 1970 to 1972 in *Science* (Wallace 1970), the *American Journal of Physiology*, and *Scientific American*. Since then more than 500 studies on TM have been conducted at 210 universities and research centers in 30 countries around the world and results have been published in more than 100 academic journals. The research on Transcendental Meditation has been collected in a single five volume publication (Orme-Johnson & Farrow 1976, Chalmers et al 1990a, 1990b, 1990c, Wallace et al 1991).

Today, after so many studies of TM have been published in peer review journals, it is not unusual to find a cardiologist or general practitioner recommending TM to patients as a way of controlling stress. This would seem a clear-cut triumph for proponents of TM, and in a way it is.

However, MAV sees TM not as just stress reduction, but as the most important way to enliven one's direct connection with the unified field, through the regular experience of the state of pure consciousness. Is there any scientific support for this more ambitious concept of Transcendental Meditation? The research bears on the question.

TRANSCENDENTAL MEDITATION AND RELAXATION

It might seem that all relaxation is alike, but the research on TM over the last decades shows something quite different. Most relaxation leads to sleepiness and dullness. By contrast, many of the studies found that TM, while producing deep physical relaxation, also simultaneously increased mental alertness.

This was Dr Wallace's original finding; in the decades since, the understanding has become more refined. In the early days of TM research, there was much focus on the total amount of oxygen the body used during meditation. If you relax, the theory goes, you burn less oxygen. Relaxation seemingly equates with less oxygen consumption. In the first studies on TM, and on other relaxation and meditation techniques invented by medical investigators, there were reports of lowered overall oxygen consumption.

As the research effort went forward, however, measuring equipment improved and research designs became more rigorous. With more rigorous testing, oxygen consumption turned out to be not such a clear-cut marker of the meditation experience. The amount of oxygen consumed during meditation was found to be highly variable, both from person to person and from experiment to experiment. In some controlled studies on Transcendental Meditation, the rate of oxygen consumption dropped significantly more than it does in eyes-closed rest; but in other studies it stayed the same. A number of other studies found that heart rate, too, did not always drop significantly more than in eyes-closed rest.

At this point, some researchers abandoned their studies. They assumed that if oxygen consumption and heart rate were not reliable measures of meditation, then meditation did not produce significant rest or relaxation. They wrote meditation off.

Several labs, however, pressed forward with the research. At the University of California (Irvine) Medical Center, Dr A.F. Wilson, the Chief of Pulmonary Medicine, worked with his colleague, Dr Ronald Jevning, and others on a series of detailed studies comparing people practicing the Transcendental Meditation technique with others sitting with eyes closed. Dr Wilson does not meditate himself, but he was intrigued by some unusual findings his team made in their early investigations.

One thing they found was that during TM metabolism in arm muscles dropped significantly; there was no change in the control group (Jevning et al 1983). This indicated that the body's musculature was relaxing. Wilson and Jevning also found that, in blood withdrawn while subjects meditated, red blood cells showed reduced metabolism (Jevning & Wilson 1977). This was a highly unusual finding. Ordinarily, red blood cells do not slow down even during sleep. Floating in the bloodstream, they have no direct connection with the operation of the nervous system; their metabolism ordinarily remains constant 24 hours a day. Finally, the team found that during TM blood flow to the arms and legs, and also to the internal organs, decreased markedly (Jevning et al 1976). During ordinary rest, blood flow to the internal organs *increases* (thus encouraging digestion, for example).

Dr Wilson's team faced two puzzles. First, their studies had shown that during Transcendental Meditation there was a clear pattern of physical rest and relaxation – reduced metabolism in muscles and blood cells – even if earlier studies on overall oxygen consumption had been ambiguous. Second, blood flow decreased to extremities and internal organs, but the heart rate did not slow down. Both puzzles came down to one: If the heart is still pumping normally, where does the missing blood go?

The group hypothesized that, during TM, there must be a significant increase in blood flow to the brain. People who practice Transcendental Meditation report feeling more alert and awake than usual.

Maharishi maintains that Transcendental Meditation improves the quality of consciousness. Perhaps increased blood flow to the brain supplies oxygen and nutrients for increased brain cell activity, while at the same time keeping the heart rate and overall oxygen consumption relatively normal.

The study was done, and the hypothesis proved correct. There was a marked increase in cerebral blood flow (Jevning & Wilson 1978). A completely new pattern of physiological activity had been discovered: overall physiological rest and relaxation combined with an enriched blood supply to the brain.

BRAIN WAVES

A similar refinement took place in the understanding of how Transcendental Meditation affects the EEG. Early researchers assumed that the relaxed state produced by Transcendental Meditation must simply involve increased alpha wave activity. It did indeed: during Transcendental Meditation, there is a marked increase in alpha power in the frontal region of the brain, a much greater increase than occurs in eyes-closed resting (Wallace 1970, Banquet 1973). Such brain waves indicate a relaxed but alert style of functioning. But some form of alpha waves can be produced by many techniques, such as biofeedback. If alpha was all that Transcendental Meditation produced, it was interesting, but didn't seem to support the idea that something unique happened in TM.

Again, though, later researchers found that there was more to it. Levine (1976), Banquet (1973), Orme-Johnson (1977), Orme-Johnson & Haynes (1981), and Badawi et al (1984), found that the most significant brain-wave marker of Transcendental Meditation involves the *overall pattern* of brain waves. The EEG signals from the different areas of the brain are usually distinct, but during Transcendental Meditation they show what are called 'stable phase relations' – that is, they become synchronized. (Technically, this was measured by Fourier analysis of the brain waves; if the resulting sine waves attained correlations of over 0.95, they were counted as being coherent; see Levine 1976) What was most interesting about this finding was that the EEG coheres in the frontal and central regions of the brain. This is a pattern of brain-wave coherence never previously seen.

COMPARATIVE RESEARCH ON MEDITATION

The above findings showed that Transcendental Meditation produces a state very different from normal rest. This conclusion was further supported by a comparative study done by Drs Michael Dillbeck and David Orme-Johnson at Maharishi International University (now Maharishi University of Management) in Fairfield, Iowa. The two psychologists attempted to produce a thorough examination of research on meditation that could be repeated by any other scholar, and that would define it as definitively as possible.

They began their work with a literature search, and found 31 scientific papers previously conducted at many universities and research institutes. Each study took measurements on people during Transcendental Meditation and/or on people sitting with eyes closed. Using a standard mathematical procedure called meta-analysis, Drs Dillbeck and Orme-Johnson produced a statistical comparison. Such a meta-analysis is considered more accurate than an individual study by itself, because it compares data from an extensive group of subjects. Also, a meta-analysis is completely objective; other researchers can undertake their own literature search and replicate the statistical analysis.

The study showed that, on several parameters, Transcendental Meditation produced a level of rest much deeper than eyes-closed rest:

1. During Transcendental Meditation the autonomic nervous system became much more stable than during eyes-closed rest, as measured by significantly higher basal skin resistance ($p < 0.05$).
2. The rate of respiration during Transcendental Meditation slowed down significantly more ($p < 0.05$) than in eyes-closed rest (even though total oxygen consumption and heart rate were not significantly lower).
3. Compared to the resting control groups, the Transcendental Meditation subjects showed a much larger ($p < 0.01$) decrease in plasma lactate, a chemical marker of metabolic activity.

The study concluded that Transcendental Meditation produces a unique pattern of physiological relaxation, clearly deeper than rest during simple eyes-closed resting (Dillbeck & Orme-Johnson 1987).

A FOURTH STATE OF CONSCIOUSNESS

On the basis of findings like those of Wallace, Wilson, Jevning, Orme-Johnson, and Dillbeck, and the EEG studies, many researchers now feel that the distinctive change in physiological functioning during Transcendental Meditation confirms Maharishi's description of TM producing a fourth major state of consciousness. It is well known that during the three common states of consciousness – waking, sleeping, and dreaming – the body functions in three completely different ways. For every state of consciousness, there is a distinctly different style of physical functioning. To many researchers, Transcendental Meditation, viewed in detail, paints a picture of a totally new style of physiological functioning. There are many signs of deep relaxation – reduced muscle and red blood cell metabolism, more stable nervous system functioning (Orme-Johnson 1977), reduced levels of cortisol (a biochemical marker of stress) and plasma lactate, and reduced breath rate (Jevning et al 1983). At the same time, blood flow to the brain increases in a highly distinctive way, and a unique pattern of frontal and central brain-wave coherence occurs. Overall, this pattern of functioning is completely different from the patterns seen in waking, sleeping and dreaming.

CLINICAL VALUE OF EXPERIENCING THE FOURTH STATE

TM, then, seems clearly to involve more than just stress reduction; it seems to produce, as Maharishi had explained from the outset, a fourth major state of consciousness. What is important for clinicians, though, is the clinical applicability of this fourth state of consciousness. According to the MAV model, it should have significant clinical value, since MAV views experiencing Transcendental Consciousness as the single most important strategy for both prevention and cure.

Further scientific research has provided a considerable amount of data consistent with the theory that regular experience of Transcendental Consciousness has significant health benefits, and that they involve a wide range of areas of life. These also bear on the question of whether Transcendental Meditation is just relaxation, or is something more.

TRANSCENDENTAL MEDITATION AND ANXIETY

Since the 1970s, when research on Transcendental Meditation began to appear, many other meditation and stress management techniques have been invented and scientifically studied. It has often been said that all of these techniques reduce stress with about equal effectiveness. But this is a question that can be and has been studied in statistical detail in a meta-analysis. In this exhaustive study, nearly two decades of stress-related studies were compared statistically, with the results printed in the *Journal of Clinical Psychology* (Eppley et al 1989).

The original studies used in this meta-analysis measured anxiety as an emotional sign of stress. Because meditation and relaxation techniques are supposed to reduce stress, psychologists have tested their effects on anxiety more than on any other parameter.

Dr Kenneth Eppley, a researcher at SRI International (formerly Stanford Research Institute), decided to do a search for such anxiety studies; he found more than 100. These studies tested the effectiveness of every well-known meditation and relaxation technique, including Transcendental Meditation, other types of meditation, the much-researched progressive muscle relaxation technique, the relaxation response (which uses the sound 'one' or other self-chosen sounds as mantras), and many others. Using the statistical methods of meta-analysis, Eppley compared all the techniques. The results challenged the common perception that all meditation and relaxation techniques are equally effective. In the results of all the tests together, the Transcendental Meditation technique reduced anxiety more than twice as much as any other technique ($p < 0.005$).

Dr Eppley had enough studies available to allow some important breakdowns in the statistical data. One of the most important of these breakdowns looked at those studies with strong research designs.

In any new field of research, it is typical that the first research – usually pilot studies – are fairly simple tests to see if results are produced and if more research is warranted. These first studies are, of course, often done quickly and inexpensively, with less-than-rigorous research designs. For instance, they may be done with only one-time testing, rather than pre- and posttesting with a time lag in between. They may not be funded enough to allow the use of a large number of subjects. They may not have a control group, which makes it harder to rule out alternative explanations for the findings. If they do have a control group, they may not use random assignment to the control group, which means that people can 'self-select' into the experimental and control groups, and self-selected subjects may bring biases and predispositions with them. Even with control groups, there may be a large dropout rate among test subjects before the study ends, which can seriously bias the results. For example, if all the most anxious people drop out of the study, leaving only the less anxious people to take the final test, the post-test would show less anxiety even if the meditation technique itself had no effect.

These issues have often been raised with meditation research. In the 1970s, many initial studies on all techniques were pilot studies. It is possible to say that the positive results from some of these studies might have been due to inadequacies in research design. According to this criticism, researchers who were biased toward a specific meditation or relaxation technique might get results they wanted if the studies were not rigorous enough.

Dr Eppley was in a position to answer such questions. First, he analyzed all the results to see which aspects of research design actually made a difference in this body of research. He found two factors most significant: random assignment to control groups and dropout rate (known as attrition). From the overall group of more than 100 studies, he then chose only those studies that had both random assignment and low attrition. All these studies had been published in academic journals or conducted as doctoral dissertations under the guidance of academic experts.

The results of this comparison did show that more stringent research design deflated results for most techniques. In studies using rigorous methodologies, most techniques reduced anxiety only 50% as deeply as they had when all studies, regardless of the rigor of their design, had been considered. In other words, these techniques had seemed to be more effective in the weaker studies than they actually turned out to be when investigated in more rigorous studies. With the Transcendental Meditation technique, however, the results held steady. Indeed, in the well-designed stud-

ies, the reduction of anxiety by Transcendental Meditation was slightly greater. Transcendental Meditation had reduced anxiety twice as much as other techniques when all studies were considered; when Dr Eppley restricted his analysis to only the best studies, Transcendental Meditation reduced anxiety more than four times as well as all the other techniques.

Because Transcendental Meditation was the first technique to be scientifically tested and has always received the most publicity, its research has always received the most scrutiny. For this reason, Eppley next made a selection of only those studies that were (1) well designed and (2) had been done by researchers who were either neutral or actively hostile toward Transcendental Meditation. He wanted only those studies that were both rigorous and clearly objective. The results indicated conclusively that the stress-reducing effects of Transcendental Meditation were not the result of experimenter bias. In this selection of studies by neutral researchers, the Transcendental Meditation technique was found to reduce anxiety about 20% more effectively than it did in all the studies taken together.

TRANSCENDENTAL MEDITATION, STRESS, AND FREE RADICALS

The effectiveness of Transcendental Meditation in anxiety reduction should have broader health implications. These have also emerged in various studies. One involves what are known as free radicals – a topic we will discuss in considerable detail in Chapter 8 on herbal remedies.

To introduce the topic briefly, many of us tend to think of oxygen as the most benign element imaginable, but in fact, it has a dark side. Various metabolic processes create highly reactive forms of oxygen and other molecules; these are the 'free radicals'. These unstable molecules eat away at other molecules. Although free radicals serve as part of our defense against invading pathogens, they also can cause extensive damage to our own cells, including to our DNA.

It might seem as though free radical damage ought to be a rare, marginal occurrence, but this is far from the case. Free radical damage has been implicated in up to 80% of all human diseases, including atherosclerosis, cancer, heart disease, inflammatory diseases, degenerative diseases, and Alzheimer's. More generally, free radicals may cause much of the general deterioration of mind and body associated with aging.

Researchers have identified a number of factors that generate excess free radicals, including mental stress, pollution, excessive sun exposure, overexertion, radiation, chemotherapy, and ingestion of alcohol, tobacco, meat, and smoked, barbecued, or processed foods. Reducing these factors will reduce the level of free radicals, also called 'oxidants', and thus improve health. Since Transcendental Meditation is remarkably effective in reducing stress, it might be expected to reduce free radical generation.

By 'stress' we mean not environmental challenges themselves, but how our body reacts to them. The stress syndrome, or fight-or-flight response, was designed to deal with prehistoric emergencies, which were of short duration and called for quick reactions. It serves us ill in the post-industrial age, where most of our emergencies are slow-burn aggravations – traffic jams or irate bosses who plague day-to-day existence. The body reacts to these with what amounts to neurochemical overkill. And many of the specific processes involved – the generation of cortisol and other stress-related chemicals and even the basic increase in energy creation involved in the stress response – greatly increase free radical production. In a variety of ways, stress causes the body to produce its own toxic substances, the free radicals.

Does Transcendental Meditation, then, with its ability to counter stress, reduce free radical production? Research shows that it does. A study done by one of the authors (Sharma) at Ohio State, with Dr Robert Schneider and other collaborators at Maharishi University of Management, compared elderly long-term meditators to controls matched for age (Sharma 1993). It looked at lipid peroxide levels. Lipid peroxides are fats that have been damaged by free radicals, and that in turn can cause a great deal of damage of their own. They are used to assess free radical levels, because it is assumed that if lipid peroxide levels are high (the result of free radical damage to lipids), free radical levels must be high. Another factor might be how much fat the person consumes, but the fat content of both the TM and the control groups' diets had been the same for years in this experiment. Yet the media-

tors showed significantly lower levels of lipid peroxides. Those between ages 60 and 69 showed 14.5% lower levels, and those between ages 70 and 79 showed 16.5% lower (Sharma 1993). This magnitude of reduction is about what one would want, since a certain level of free radicals is necessary for the body's self-defense, and the body's own antioxidant and repair mechanisms can handle excess free radicals up to a certain point.

TRANSCENDENTAL MEDITATION AND AGING

A number of studies, using very different approaches, have found Transcendental Meditation to reverse or slow the aging process.

The first study on this topic was done by Wallace, the pioneer of meditation research. He used the Adult Growth Examination, a test derived in part from the United States National Health Survey, standardized using a carefully selected representative cross-sample of several thousand adults, and validated in various studies in North America (Morgan & Fevens 1972). The examination measures basic functions – including near-point vision, auditory discrimination, and blood pressure – that typically decline with age. This test helped lead to the concept of biological age as distinct from chronological age. Biological age measures age in terms of physical function; chronological age measures age in terms of years. George Bernard Shaw died at the age of 94 years as the result of injuries sustained when he fell from a tree he was pruning. He probably had a biological age much younger than his chronological age up until his final days.

Dr Wallace applied the test to 73 people between the ages of 40 and 64 years who practice Transcendental Meditation. His study statistically controlled for the effects of diet and exercise. As compared to normal values established over many years, those who had practiced Transcendental Meditation for up to 5 years had an average biological age 5 years younger than their chronological age. Those who had meditated for more than 5 years had an average biological age 12 years younger (Wallace et al 1982).

Wallace's study has since been corroborated by other studies. In a study published in the *Journal of Behavioral Medicine*, Dr Jay Glaser (Glaser et al 1992) looked at hormonal markers of aging. Aging is partially caused by a reduction in hormone secretion. Without certain hormones, the body withers. Richard Cutler has theorized that reduced hormonal secretions may be due to cell dysdifferentiation (cells 'forget' what they are specialized to do, and behave in a more general manner), and that this is caused by free radical damage (Cutler 1985). The same effect could be caused by atherosclerosis in the blood vessels leading to the hypothalamus, pituitary, and other glands – and free radical damage plays a critical role in this process. If stress creates free radicals, and free radical damage reduces the level of hormones, then Transcendental Meditation should serve to maintain high levels of such hormones.

Glaser tested this by looking at one of the body's most significant hormones – dehydroepiandrosterone sulfate (DHEA-S). In a young adult, DHEA-S is the most abundant hormone in the body, but the levels decline rapidly with age. Men who maintain relatively high levels of DHEA-S have been shown to have less atherosclerosis and heart disease, and lower mortality rate from all causes. Women with high levels of DHEA-S are known to have less breast cancer and osteoporosis. Whereas the stress hormone cortisol leads to the breakdown of muscle tissue (to provide fuel for energy), DHEA-S leads to the build-up of muscle tissue. Influenced by DHEA-S, the body continues to build, instead of wasting away.

The study compared DHEA-S levels in the blood of 423 people who practiced Transcendental Meditation to the levels of 1253 who did not. The ages ranged from 20 to 81 years. Results were gathered in 5-year age ranges. The effects of diet, obesity, and exercise were statistically ruled out. The results were consistent with Wallace's study. Depending on the age range, people who practiced Transcendental Meditation had levels of DHEA-S that were as high as members of the control group who were 5 to 10 years younger (Glaser et al 1992).

Also relevant is Smith et al's (1989) finding that TM practitioners had a significantly lower blood erythrocyte sedimentation rate (ESR) than matched controls – which included a large group of vegetarian monks and nuns practicing a meditative lifestyle and a group of Seventh Day Adventists. ESR rates are correlated with aging and premature mortality.

A COMPARISON STUDY OF THE ELDERLY

Another corroboration of Wallace's study came from a Harvard University study of 77 elderly nursing home residents. This study, conducted by the psychologists Charles N. Alexander and Ellen K. Langer, compared three types of meditation and relaxation techniques – TM, 'mindfulness training' and 'mental relaxation', a meditation technique loosely modeled on Transcendental Meditation but involving no mantra, but rather any sound the participant found pleasant. There was also a no-treatment control group. The residents, with an average age of 81 years, were randomly assigned to the four groups. The study, which lasted 3 years altogether, showed that residents in the Transcendental Meditation group had the greatest reductions in stress ($p < 0.01$) and blood pressure ($p < 0.01$). The Transcendental Meditation group also had a significantly higher survival rate ($p < 0.00025$): they were the only group in which no one died during the study, although the average mortality rate in non-participating residents during those 3 years was more than one-third (Table 3.1). Interestingly, the 'mental relaxation' technique, supposedly modeled on TM, had the highest mortality rate and highest blood pressure and the least improvement in mental health: their results in survival rate and blood pressure were *worse* than the control group's (Alexander et al 1989).

Some years later, the researchers did a follow up study of the above groups, and found that the results held up. After 8 years, the Transcendental Meditation group's mean survival time was 65% higher than that of the other groups combined; after 15 years, it was 22% higher. Cardiovascular and all-cause mortality showed a similar pattern: the TM group had distinct decreases compared to the other groups (Alexander et al 1996).

Table 3.1 Survival rates among experimental and control groups of elderly nursing home residents

Technique	% still living after 36 months
TM	100
Mindfulness	87.5
Relaxation	65
No treatment	77.3

CLINICAL RESULTS

Does Transcendental Meditation, then, actually create better health? Here the research findings are voluminous. Studies on specific health risk factors – such as cholesterol (Cooper & Aygen 1978, 1979), cardiovascular disease (Zamarra et al 1996), smoking (Alexander et al 1994b) – have all shown Transcendental Meditation to have highly significant benefits. For example, in a controlled, randomized study, published in *Hypertension* in 1995, Schneider et al randomly assigned 128 elderly African-American hypertensives to groups practicing Transcendental Meditation, progressive muscle relaxation, or diet and exercise. Over a 3 month period, the reductions in blood pressure were significantly greater for the TM group than for the other two (Table 3.2).

This finding – that TM produced significantly greater reductions in hypertension than progressive muscle relaxation – is congruent with a meta-analysis of various techniques *other than TM*, such as Benson's 'relaxation response' technique, biofeedback, non-TM meditations, and progressive muscle relaxation. Their effects on hypertension were found to be no greater than that of placebo techniques (Eisenberg et al 1993). By contrast, a number of studies have found TM to reduce hypertension significantly compared to controls (Cooper & Aygen 1978, Alexander et al 1989, Schneider et al 1992, Wallace et al 1983, Kuchera 1987).

Another risk factor that TM is known to reduce is substance abuse. A special 1994 double issue of *Alcoholism Treatment Quarterly* contained 17 articles on the effectiveness of TM in this area. One article was a meta-analysis of 19 studies on TM and substance abuse (Alexander et al 1994b). Among those studies that looked at TM and substance abuse in the general population, this meta-analysis found the effect size for the TM groups to be 0.42 for alcohol and 0.74 for drug abuse (note that an effect size of 0.20 is considered

small, 0.50 to be medium, and 0.80 to be large). In populations being treated for substance abuse, the effect size for TM was greater: 1.35 for alcohol and 1.16 for illicit drugs. To get a sense of how significant these numbers are, note that a meta-analysis of the popular DARE (Drug Abuse Resistance Education) program, which is used in high schools around the country, found an effect size of only 0.06 (Ennett et al 1994). A meta-analysis also looked at 143 adolescent drug prevention programs, and found their average effect size to be only 0.17 for alcohol and 0.21 for drugs (Tobler 1986; see Marcus 1996, pp. 89–103, for a discussion).

REDUCED HEALTH CARE COSTS

Perhaps the most dramatic research on the health benefits of Transcendental Meditation looked at health insurance statistics. The first such study was published in *Psychosomatic Medicine* (Orme-Johnson 1987). Over a 5-year period, this study tracked 2000 people all across the country who practiced Transcendental Meditation. The data was collected by the insurance company. The statistics from the meditation group were compared to those of a control group selected by the insurance company to match the Transcendental Meditation group for age, education, profession, and other variables.

The overall result was that, compared to the control group, the Transcendental Meditation group went to the hospital 56% less often for illness or surgery. Although the differences between controls and the TM group were significant in all age groups, they were most pronounced in the older age groups. In addition, the TM group needed 50% fewer doctors' visits. The Transcendental Meditation group did use medical care just as much as controls only in one health arena, maternity.

The statistics in this study were gathered by the insurance company, and can be considered reliable. None the less, the study could be criticized for not being 'prospective': it did not look at people before and after. In theory, the Transcendental Meditation group may have been healthier even before they started to meditate.

To control for this, Robert Herron of MIU, now Maharishi University of Management, in a study published in the *American Journal of Health Promotion*

Table 3.2 Effects of Transcendental Meditation, progressive muscle relaxation (PMR) and diet and exercise on systolic blood pressure (SBP) and diastolic blood pressure (DBP) in randomly assigned elderly African-Americans (from Schneider et al 1995)

	Transcendental Meditation	PMR group	Diet and exercise group
SBP	−10.7	−4	−1.4
DBP	−5.9	−2.1	+0.6

(Herron et al 1996), compared medical costs in a group of 677 enrollees in the Quebec provincial health-care plan for 3 years before and after learning TM. Because Canada has national cradle-to-grave health-care coverage, the government has data on every health-care cost incurred by every citizen. It was possible to trace people's records back years before they learned Transcendental Meditation, then look for any changes. The study also was significant in that it looked not only at health-care utilization, but also at actual health-care costs. Prior to this study, no research project had found a program that could reduce health-care costs over the long term. Some programs help to contain costs, but bringing them down on a sustainable basis had been elusive.

This study found that in the years before the subjects learned TM, their health-care costs were the same as for people in their age range. They were not a self-selected group of outstandingly healthy people. Once they began to meditate, however, their health-care costs began to decline – an average of 5 to 7% each year.

The reductions were most dramatic among people who had previously shown the highest pattern of health-care costs. The total group was divided into thirds, and in the third which had been to doctors and the hospital most frequently the practice of Transcendental Meditation reduced health-care costs by 18% a year – 54% in three years. Since these declines were inflation-adjusted, the actual cost reductions were much greater.

The study did have methodological limitations, though these seem to us to be far from debilitating. It did not control for self-selection in other areas besides prior health (in which there was no difference between groups), or for changes in lifestyle or diet that TM meditators might have made in addition to starting TM (though if TM itself had caused them to make some of these healthful changes, as some studies suggest, the issue would be complicated), or for non-physician health costs (although, since these would be paid out of pocket and physician costs are paid by the state, they may not have been significant). The study did, however, control for age and gender, which in Quebec had been shown to be the best predictors of medical use and expense, and for experimenter expectation (since it was retrospective).

IS TRANSCENDENTAL MEDITATION JUST RELAXATION?

Exhaustive meta-analysis and pre-post-test random assignment comparisons are the most effective tool available for judging whether Transcendental Meditation is just relaxation, or something more. Consider the Eppley meta-analysis of anxiety and various meditation techniques, discussed above. In this case, TM, which produces a fourth state of consciousness, reduces stress and anxiety much more effectively than any other techniques tested to date. Many researchers feel that meditation is simply relaxation, but the data indicate that a fourth state of consciousness reduces anxiety two to four times better than physical relaxation techniques. Similarly, the Transcendental Meditation group in the Alexander and Langer experiment with the elderly had by far the highest survival rate of three groups doing meditation techniques, and the greatest reduction of blood pressure and stress; while one of the other techniques, designed to mimic TM, had *worse* outcomes than even the control group. The Schneider experiment found, similarly, that TM reduced hypertension more than twice as much as progressive muscle relaxation. It appears that relaxation is *not* the single active ingredient in Transcendental Meditation.

Similar studies and meta-studies have found TM to be far more effective than other techniques in bringing improvement on several other variables such as self-actualization (Alexander et al 1991, Alexander et al 1994a, Alexander et al 1994b). All these studies raise the question of why a difference might exist between techniques. An explanation suggested by the MAV viewpoint may be that the crucial factor is not meditation or stress reduction per se, but experiencing the fourth state of consciousness, transcendental consciousness. MAV would explain this by saying that, in the state of transcendental consciousness, the unity underlying diversity is fully experienced, and 'remembering' the unified field is said to enliven the patterns that should prevail in a healthy mind and body. Is there any scientific basis to this more ambitious concept of Transcendental Meditation?

There is some evidence that the experience of transcendental consciousness involves what physics calls a *field effect* – that is, that during TM the mind is connecting to a field that goes beyond the boundaries of the individual meditator's brain and spreads throughout a population. We will review this research in the final chapter of this book, but for now let us note that several published studies have shown that when a small group practices the Transcendental Meditation and the advanced TM-Sidhi program in a group, it reduces crime and violence in the population as a whole, even though the population has no obvious interaction with the group. Some ingenious ways of testing this hypothesis have produced some very significant results. This may remind you of the quantum phenomena we talked about in Chapter 2, in which the manifested world around us turns out to be waves on an underlying quantum field. Could a quantum level of the brain be involved in this phenomenon? While the brain is not generally believed to operate in a quantum mechanical way, some distinguished scientists, notably Henry Stapp, the Nobel Laureate Sir John Eccles and the Wolf Prize-winning Oxford physicist Roger Penrose, have argued that the brain does have some quantum mechanical operation (Stapp 1993,

Penrose 1994). Some sort of quantum brain behavior would lend support to the MAV view of transcendental consciousness as experience of the unified field of all the laws of nature, and help explain the research on collective effects of meditation.

TRANSCENDENTAL MEDITATION IN MAV

MAV practitioners recommend TM as an adjunct to whatever other measures they prescribe. TM is not all one would prescribe in every case, and is not necessarily what is needed to cure a specific complaint. But as a general health measure, both in the preventive and the healing stages, it is unequalled. Prescribing it is a matter, it can be argued, of common sense.

There are, in fact, other mental techniques in Maharishi's Vedic Approach to Health: advanced techniques of TM for experienced practitioners, and an advanced program called the TM-Sidhi program, which is meant to develop the ability to operate from within the unified field. We will discuss this in the final chapter of this book.

REFERENCES

Alexander C, Barnes V, Schneider R et al 1996 A randomized controlled trial of stress reduction on cardiovascular and all-cause mortality in the elderly: results of 8 year and 15 year follow ups. Circulation 93(3) (abstract)

Alexander C N, Langer E J, Davies J L, Chandler H M, Newman R I 1989 Transcendental Meditation, mindfulness, and longevity: an experimental study with the elderly. Journal of Personality and Social Psychology 57(6):950–964

Alexander C N, Rainforth M V, Gelderloos P 1991 Transcendental Meditation, self-actualization, and psychological health: a conceptual overview and statistical meta-analysis. Journal of Social Behavior and Personality 6(5):189–247

Alexander C N, Robinson P, Orme-Johnson D W, Schneider R H, Walton K G 1994a The effects of Transcendental Meditation compared to other methods of relaxation and meditation in reducing risk factors, morbidity, and mortality. Homeostasis 35:243–264

Alexander C N, Robinson P, Rainforth M 1994b Treating and preventing alcohol, nicotine, and drug abuse through Transcendental Meditation: a review and statistical meta-analysis. Alcoholism Treatment Quarterly 11:11–84

Badawi K, Wallace R K, Orme-Johnson D W, Rouzere A M 1984 Electrophysiologic characteristics of respiratory suspension periods during the practice of the Transcendental Meditation program. Psychosomatic Medicine 46:267–276

Banquet J P 1973 Spectral analysis of the EEG in meditation. Electroencephalography and Clinical Neurophysiology 35:145–151

Chalmers R, Clements G, Schenkluhn H, Weinless M 1990a Scientific research on Maharishi's Transcendental Meditation

program: collected papers. Maharishi European Research University Press, Seelisberg, Switzerland, vol 2

Chalmers R, Clements G, Schenkluhn H, Weinless M 1990b Scientific research on Maharishi's Transcendental Meditation program: collected papers. Maharishi European Research University Press, Vlodrop, Netherlands, vol 3

Chalmers R, Clements G, Schenkluhn H, Weinless M 1990c Scientific research on Maharishi's Transcendental Meditation program: collected papers. Maharishi European Research University Press, Vlodrop, Netherlands, vol 4

Cooper M J, Aygen M M 1978 Effect of Transcendental Meditation on serum cholesterol and blood pressure. Harefuah, the Journal of the Israel Medical Association 95(1):1–2

Cooper M J, Aygen M M 1979 A relaxation technique in the management of hypercholesterolemia. Journal of Human Stress 5:24–27

Cutler R 1985. Dysdifferentiation and aging. In: Sohal R S (ed) Molecular biology of aging: gene stability and gene expression. Raven Press, New York, 307–340

Dillbeck M C, Orme-Johnson D W 1987 Physiological differences between Transcendental Meditation and rest. American Physiologist 42:879–881

Eisenberg D M, Dilbanco T L, Berkey C S, et al 1993 Cognitive behavioral techniques for hypertension: are they effective? Annals of Internal Medicine 118(12):964–972

Ennett S T, Tobler N, Ringwalt C L, Flewelling R L 1994 How effective is Drug Abuse Resistance Education? A meta-analysis of Project DARE outcome evaluations. American Journal of Public Health 84(9):1394

Eppley K, Abrams A, Shear J 1989 Differential effects of relaxation techniques on trait anxiety: a meta-analysis. Journal of Clinical Psychology, 45(6):957–974

Glaser J L, Brind J L, Vogelman J H et al 1992 Elevated serum dehydroepiandrosterone-sulfate levels in practitioners of the Transcendental Meditation (TM) and TM-Sidhi programs. Journal of Behavioral Medicine 15(4):327–341

Herron R E, Hillis S L, Mandarino J V, Orme-Johnson D W, Walton K G 1996 The impact of the Transcendental Meditation program on government payments to physicians in Quebec. American Journal of Health Promotion 10(3):208–216

Jevning R, Smith R, Wilson AF, Morton M E 1976 Alterations in blood flow during Transcendental Meditation. Psychophysiology 13:168(abstract)

Jevning R, Wilson A F 1977 Altered red cell metabolism in TM. Psychophysiology 14:94(abstract)

Jevning R, Wilson A F 1978 Behavioral increase of cerebral blood flow. The Physiologist 21:60

Jevning R, Wilson F, O'Halloran J P, Walsh R N 1983 Forearm blood flow and metabolism during stylized and unstylized states of decreased activation. American Journal of Physiology 245 (Regul Integr Comp Physiol 14):R110–116

Kuchera M M 1987 The effectiveness of meditation techniques to reduce blood pressure levels: a meta-analysis. Dissertation Abstracts International 57:4639B

Levine J P 1976 The Coherence Spectral Array (COSPAR) and its application to the study of spatial ordering in the EEG. Proceedings of the San Diego Biomedical Symposium 15:237–247

Marcus J B 1996 The crime vaccine. Claitor, Baton Rouge

Morgan R F, Fevens S K 1972 Reliability of the adult growth examination: a standardized test of individual aging. Perceptual and Motor Skills 34:415–419

Orme-Johnson D W 1977 EEG coherence during transcendental consciousness. Electroencephalography and Clinical Neurophysiology 43(4):581–582,E 487 (abstract)

Orme-Johnson D W 1987 Medical care utilization and the Transcendental Meditation program. Psychosomatic Medicine 49:493–507

Orme-Johnson D W, Farrow J T 1976 Scientific research on the Transcendental Meditation program: collected papers. Maharishi European Research University Press, Seelisberg, Switzerland, vol 1

Orme-Johnson D W, Haynes C T 1981 EEG phase coherence, pure

consciousness, creativity, and the TM-Sidhi experience. International Journal of Neuroscience 113:211–219

Penrose R 1994 Shadows of the mind. Oxford University Press, Oxford, pp 348–352

Schneider R H, Alexander C N, Wallace R K 1992 In search of an optimal behavioral treatment for hypertension: a review and focus on Transcendental Meditation. In: Johnson E H, Gentry W D, Julius S (eds) Personality, elevated blood pressure, and essential hypertension. Hemisphere, Washington, DC, pp. 291–316

Schneider R H, Staggers F, Alexander C N et al 1995 A randomized controlled trial of stress reduction for hypertension in older African Americans. Hypertension 26(5):820–837

Sharma H M 1993 Freedom from disease. Veda, Toronto, pp 186–188

Smith D E, Glaser J L, Schneider R H, Dillbeck M C 1989 Erythrocyte sedimentation rate (ESR) and the Transcendental Meditation (TM) program. Psychosomatic Medicine 5:259

Stapp H P 1993 Mind, matter and quantum mechanics. Springer-Verlag, Berlin

Tobler N 1986 Meta-analysis of 143 drug prevention programs: quantitative outcome results of program participants compared to a control or comparison group. Journal of Drug Issues 16:537–567

Wallace R K 1970 Physiological effects of Transcendental Meditation. Science 167:1751–1754

Wallace R K, Dillbeck M C, Jacobe E, Harrington B 1982 The effects of the Transcendental Meditation and TM-Sidhi program on the aging process. International Journal of Neuroscience 16:53–58

Wallace R K, Orme-Johnson D W, Dillbeck M C 1991 Scientific research on Maharishi's Transcendental Meditation Program: collected papers. Maharishi International University Press, Fairfield, Iowa, vol 5

Wallace R K, Silver J, Mills P, Dillbeck M C, Wagner D E 1983 Systolic blood pressure and long-term practice of the Transcendental Meditation and TM-Sidhi program: effects of TM on blood pressure. Psychosomatic Medicine 45:41–46

Zamarra J W, Schneider R H, Besseghini I, Robinson D K, Salerno J W 1996 Usefulness of the Transcendental Meditation program in the treatment of patients with coronary artery disease. American Journal of Cardiology 77:867–870

4

The effect of emotions and thinking on health

Maharishi Ayur-Veda (MAV)'s model of health is based on consciousness – that field which lies beneath thinking and feeling – but it hardly neglects the influence of thought and emotion on health.

A generation ago, MAV's idea that behaviors and emotions could affect health profoundly would have seemed dubious to most medical scientists; even a decade ago, the *New England Journal of Medicine* characterized the idea that emotions influence disease as 'folklore'. Today this is a medical commonplace. Numerous studies have found links between the two, and most people have heard of the anecdotal evidence that popularized the idea, such as the story of Norman Cousins, who overcame a life-threatening disease by watching Marx Brothers movies and otherwise maintaining a happy mood.

HOW BEHAVIOR AND EMOTION INFLUENCE HEALTH: *OJAS* AND THE THREE *GUNAS*

The essential way in which the MAV 'consciousness' model explains the effects of mind on body has already been mentioned. As we saw, consciousness, mind, and body are understood to be three parts of a continuum, with consciousness at the basis. In the sequence of manifestation, mind is an earlier manifestation than body. Thus it is to be expected that the mind will have a profound impact on the body. This is the outline; but the MAV model gives some specific details not yet covered.

We spoke before of three steps in the sequence of the manifestation of the mental sphere: ego (*ahamkara*, which literally means 'I-ness'), intellect (*buddhi*), and mind (*manas*). The I-ness is the manifestation of individuality from the universal. *Buddhi*, or intellect, is that element which discriminates. Its failure to recall the underlying unity while becoming engrossed in the sequential manifestations of diversity is called *pragya-aparadh*, the mistake of the intellect, and is said to lead to disease in a variety of ways. Then there is *manas*, the mind. The mind entertains thoughts, some health-promoting, some not. We have already seen how MAV, through Transcendental Meditation, its primary mental technique, brings full balance and integration to the *ahamkara*, intellect, and mind, and how this also has a profound impact on the physiology. But MAV supplements this with further understanding of how thoughts, the contents of mind, affect the body, and of approaches to this area that yield the best effect.

The three *gunas*

One factor MAV considers is the three *gunas*, *sattwa*, *rajas*, and *tamas*. These are said to manifest prior to matter, just as mind is said to be prior to the body. In Maharishi's definitions:

The process of evolution is carried on by these three gunas. Evolution means creation and its progressive development, and at its basis lies activity. Activity needs rajo-guna to create a spur, and it needs sato-guna and tamo-guna to uphold the direction of the movement.

The nature of tamo-guna is to check and retard, but it should not be thought that when the movement is upwards, tamo-guna is absent. For any process to continue, there have to be stages in that process, and each stage, however small in time and space, needs a force to maintain it, and another force to develop it into a new stage .... The force that develops it into a new stage is sato-guna, while tamo-guna is that which checks or retards the process in order to maintain the stage already produced so that it may form the basis for the next stage. (Maharishi Maheshi Yogi, 1966)

As this suggests, the *gunas*' influence is universal, but in terms of the human mind they have specific influences. *Sattwa*, the creative influence, is entirely positive; *rajas*, the spur to activity, and *tamas*, the retarding or inertial influence, are necessary to some degree, but beyond that degree become negative. Charaka describes people dominated by *sattwa* as 'endowed with memory, devotion; grateful, learned, pure, courageous, skillful, resolute, fighting in battles with prowess, free from anxiety, having well-directed

and serious intellect, and engaged in virtuous acts.' (*Charaka Samhita, Vimanasthanam*, VIII, 110). *Rajas*, by contrast, gives a tendency to anger and lack of self-control, and *tamas* to inertia, corruption, and dullness.

Anything which increases *sattwa* in the mind is considered highly valuable; anything which reduces it, or which increases *rajas* or *tamas*, is to be moderated. We will look below at factors that influence health; one of the ways in which they do so is by increasing *sattwa*. The behavioral *rasayanas*, discussed in this chapter, are all said to increase *sattwa*. Diet is said to have an influence: certain foods, such as rice, almonds, ghee (Ch. 7, Appendix 2), milk, and honey, increase *sattwa*. Foods that increase *rajas* include red meat, as well as food that is too salty, sour, hot, spicy, or sharp. If food leaves a burning sensation (some chilis, for example), it is increasing *rajas*. Foods that increase *tamas* include alcohol, 'junk food', and leftovers. If the food is stale, putrid, decaying, impure, or has lost its flavor, it increases *tamas*.

However, the most effective way to increase *sattwa*, according to MAV, is mental techniques to expand consciousness, notably the Transcendental Meditation and the TM-Sidhi programs.

Ojas

Another important factor is a substance called *ojas*. *Ojas* is the end-product of perfect digestion and metabolism, but it has a more profound status than that. It is also said to stand as a 'lamp at the door' between consciousness and matter, connecting them and thus ensuring that the sequence of natural law is expressed properly in the body. It is also said to nourish and sustain the various tissues (*dhatus* – see Chapter 5) of the body.

Ojas is said to pervade the body. According to Charaka, when the quantity of *ojas* diminishes too much, life itself is threatened (*Charaka Samhita, Sutrasthana*, XVII, 74). When *ojas* is present in abundance, it gives strength, immune strength, contentment, and good digestion. It is said to be the most important biochemical substance mediating the influence of consciousness on the body.

Ojas is described as a white, oily substance. There are two types of it, ordinary and superior; the superior is said to exist in eight drops in the structure described in Ayurveda as *hridaya*. We will consider what the *hridaya* might be, anatomically speaking, in a later section of this chapter.

All Ayurvedic treatment is designed to increase the abundance of *ojas* and to avoid reducing *ojas*; both aspects are considered central to restoring health and to preventing illness.

Factors said to increase *ojas*, and that are to be maximized, include:

- Consciousness. The main factor determining *ojas* production is one's level of consciousness. As the inner Self becomes more and more 'awake', one result is said to be that more *ojas* is spontaneously produced. This may in part reflect the principle that growing to enlightenment means growing in inner happiness. Happiness is the most effective means of producing *ojas*.
- Good digestion and balanced diet. MAV's advice on diet (Ch. 7) is aimed to improve *ojas* production, for *ojas* is held to be the end-product of perfect digestion and metabolism.

Two additional points are relevant. The first is that some foods directly increase *ojas*, while others decrease it. Charaka describes the qualities of *ojas*, and says that foods with those qualities, such as milk, ghee, and rice, increase *ojas*. Foods with the opposite qualities, such as alcohol, decrease the amount and quality of *ojas*. The second point is that for *ojas* production what one eats is important, but how one prepares and eats it is also significant. Food taken in an atmosphere of warmth, upliftment, and congeniality increases *ojas*. This reflects the next factor said to increase *ojas*:

- Positivity in feelings, speech, and behavior. Love, joy, and appreciation produces more *ojas* and, therefore, better immunity. This ties in well with the current findings in mind/body medicine, and may provide a way of understanding such findings.
- *Panchakarma*, or Ayurvedic purification therapy, which removes impurities from the *shrotas*, the physiological channels in the body (see Chapter 5). This is said to improve the cells' ability to take up and receive *ojas*, thus helping rejuvenate the body (see Chapter 10).
- *Rasayanas*, special Ayurvedic herbal and mineral substances. *Rasayanas* have been defined as 'that

which causes *ojas* to be produced all over'. In Chapter 8 we look at the rationale behind *rasayanas*, and at research being done on them.

Factors that diminish *ojas*, and that should be avoided, are:

- Negative emotions of any kind.
- Stress.
- Hurrying.
- Excessive exercise. The right amount of exercise varies for different individuals. The weak feeling one gets from too much exercise is said to reflect, in part, the reduction of *ojas* (see Chapter 11).
- Fasting. Moderate fasting is sometimes used in special doctor-supervised situations in Maharishi Ayur-Veda, but excess fasting can weaken the body by emaciating the bodily tissues and reducing the *ojas* which nourishes them.
- Rough or very light diet.
- Overexposure to wind and sun.
- Staying awake through much of the night. We discuss sleep cycles in Chapter 9, which deals with daily routine.
- Excessive loss of bodily fluids (such as blood).
- Overindulgence in sexual activity.
- Injury or trauma to the body.
- Alcoholic beverages.

THE LIMBIC SYSTEM

As already mentioned, *ojas* is a biochemical substance said to have a profound influence on the quality of mental and emotional life as well as physical health. This emphasis on a biochemical substance is in line with recent understandings of the biochemical mediation of emotion and its effect on the body.

The limbic area of the brain (the physiological seat of emotions), which correlates with deep emotional states, surrounds the hypothalamus, which has often been called the 'brain's brain', and is the body's central regulatory switchboard. The hypothalamus regulates temperature, thirst, hunger, blood sugar levels, growth, sleeping, and waking, and emotions such as anger and happiness. Situated just below the hypothalamus is the pituitary gland, the body's master gland, which emits secretions that control the activity of many other glands in the body. Taken together, these three elements – the limbic area, hypothalamus, and pituitary – form the 'limbic system', which alters with every alteration in emotions, creating a new mix of molecules which transform the functioning of the body.

The hypothalamus is impacted by stimuli from a number of sources: the five senses; the immune system; cognitive information; and above all, emotion. Stimuli coming from the limbic region of the brain cause the hypothalamus to release a wide variety of neuropeptides. These neuropeptides, in turn, stimulate specific hormones from the pituitary gland and, thus, specific activity in all endocrine glands, including the thymus and adrenal glands. This new combination of chemical messengers changes the operation and make-up of the body, especially the metabolic system and the immune system.

Through the action of the limbic system, particular psychological and emotional states take on molecular form. When you watch an 'action movie', you may begin to feel a nervous stomach and sweaty palms. Specific chemical messengers have been released. The body has been changed by what it is seeing on the screen. The emotions raised by the movie correlate with activity in the limbic system.

Metabolizing experience

In this sense, the body metabolizes the emotional content of every experience it has. Happiness registering in the limbic region stimulates one cascade of chemicals from the hypothalamus and pituitary, with corresponding physiological changes everywhere in the body. Sadness creates another cascade, and another physiology.

The hypothalamus can also communicate with the body directly. It modulates the activity of the autonomic nervous system. And neuropeptides produced by the hypothalamus act on the pituitary and other areas. In fact, there are receptors for them on cells throughout the body. An action movie can create a nervous stomach because the digestive tract has receptors for stress-response neuropeptides.

More significantly, these receptors have been found on immune system lymphocytes (fast-reacting immune system cells) all over the body (Faith et al 1991). Apparently, lymphocytes can tune in to the molecular messages created by thoughts and feelings. On the other hand, chemicals created by the lymphocytes, such as interleukins, have receptors in the hypothalamic region of the brain. Thus, chemical messages from the immune system can modulate nervous system functioning and mental states (Faith et al 1991). There is a two-way communication network between the brain and the immune system. A growing body of data also suggests that neurotransmitters produced by the autonomic nervous system can communicate directly with the immune system and modify its functioning (Fig. 4.1).

Ojas and the hypothalamus

Is there more than a broad analogy between modern findings regarding neuro-immuno-modulators and the Ayurvedic one? One hypothesis is that *ojas* might be equivalent to neuropeptides from the hypothalamus, which have identical effects. Also, as we said, the most important part of *ojas* is said to come from a structure called the *hridaya*. The *hridaya* is often translated as 'heart'. Some propose that the Ayurvedic texts suggest that they do not mean the circulatory pump, but something subtler; in line with the previous speculation about *ojas*, one hypothesis is that the *hridaya* may be equivalent to the hypothalamus. Admittedly, there is insufficient evidence to conclude this definitively at this point.

TRANSCENDENTAL MEDITATION REVISITED

In Chapter 3 we discussed Transcendental Meditation in terms of stress reduction, brain-wave coherence, free radicals, and, above all, transcendental experience of the unified field. TM also can be said to have an influence through the limbic system. Instead of metabolizing stress, the limbic system during Transcendental Meditation metabolizes peace and contentment. This would lead to a better character of neurochemical influence throughout the body, thus producing better health.

'BEHAVIORAL *RASAYANAS*'

Another way through which the effect of mind on

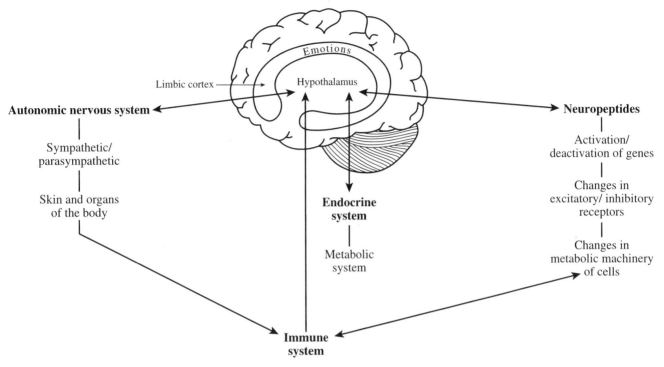

Figure 4.1   The limbic system

health is handled in MAV is through 'behavioral *rasayanas*'. *Rasayana* is MAV's term for substances that strengthen immunity (see Chapter 8). But using it to describe certain behavioral patterns seems insightful. It now is clear that the body has its own internal 'pharmacological laboratory' in the hypothalamus, pituitary, and so on – which also produce substances that influence immune strength. Neuropeptides affect the whole body: negative emotions like anger, hate, or fear release a rush of neurochemicals that strain and damage the organs; positive emotions like love, laughter, and appreciation release health-promoting chemicals. Laughter, for example, reduces levels of such stress hormones as cortisol and epinephrine, and increases the activity of immune cells, such as T cells, natural killer cells and antibodies. A positive mental state correlates with increased survival time for some patients with AIDS and cancer. Severe mental depression, by contrast, has been shown to result in suppression or even loss of immune system functioning (Hillhouse et al 1991).

The 'behavioral *rasayanas*' deal with the mind's influence on the body in a systematic way: they prescribe behaviors that elicit health-promoting biochemical effects. These are valuable both for prevention and as adjuncts to treatments. They include such traditional virtues as moderation and respect for teachers and elders, and such emotions as love and compassion. They exclude such emotions or moods as anger, negativity, and violence, which are said to damage health. One result of practicing the behavioral *rasayanas* is that the limbic system is metabolizing positive emotions far more often, and negative ones far less so.

Specific behavioral *rasayanas* mentioned in the *Charaka Samhita* and other classical Ayurvedic sources are listed in Box 4.1. Note that these are traditional teachings in many cultures; this reflects the insight of long-lived traditions into the principles upholding human health.

Charaka lists another behavioral *rasayana*: 'knowing the measure of time and place with propriety'. This refers, among other things, to what we now call chronobiology, the study of daily and annual physiological cycles. We will discuss MAV's detailed advice on this in Chapter 9.

It is significant that these teachings relate to the issue of *pragya-aparadh*; overcoming *pragya-aparadh* (mistakes of the intellect) will lead one spontaneously to uphold the behavioral *rasayanas*.

Box 4.1 Behavioral *rasayanas*

Behaviors and attitudes to be maximized:

- Love.
- Compassion.
- Speech that uplifts people.
- Cleanliness.
- Charity and regular donation.
- Religious observance.
- Respect towards teachers and elders.
- Being positive.
- Moderation and self-control, especially with regard to alcohol and sex.
- Simplicity.

To be avoided:

- Anger.
- Violence.
- Harsh or hurtful speech.
- Conceit.
- Speaking ill of others behind their backs.
- Egotism.
- Dishonesty.
- Coveting another's spouse or wealth.

BEDSIDE MANNER

Another way in which the effect of the mind on health is attended to in MAV is through what medicine has traditionally called 'bedside manner'. Family doctors were once known for their warm and reassuring bedside manner, and every good physician knew that if patients felt comforted and encouraged they would do better. Until recently, however, family doctors have been a disappearing species, and fear of a malpractice suit had led doctors to reverse their style: to tell their patients of every conceivable catastrophe their symptoms might lead to, lest they be accused of incompetence. MAV strongly encourages physicians to resist such pressures: while it is important for the patient to be informed, one should also remember that too much directness can destroy a patient's sense of well-being.

The MAV physician is aided in this regard by the use of subtle, non-invasive diagnostic procedures, the most important of which are reviewed in Chapter 6.

THE 'CONSCIOUSNESS MODEL': A SUMMARY

The last three chapters have examined part of the theoretical basis of MAV and its practical applications. The Western model has seen the body as a Newtonian machine, but the MAV model sees it as a dynamic pattern of knowledge, with its basis in the transcendental unified field. The mind/body is held in the MAV model to have, as its basis, the total potential of natural law. It is not surprising, then, that all of MAV's modalities aim to enliven the full expression of the inner intelligence of the body. We will see that aim expressed in this book when we talk about such modalities as herbs, diet, and daily routine.

The mind/body's basis is held to be a field of pure, abstract knowledge, the unified field, which MAV holds, is experienced directly as Transcendental Consciousness, which can be achieved through the practice of TM. For several reasons, this experience is said to be the most important thing one can do for promoting health. There is now substantial evidence that TM does benefit health in numerous ways; there is also a large number of studies that finds it more effective than generic meditation or stress reduction exercises, suggesting that something beyond simple stress reduction may be at work.

In addition to the revolutionary idea of consciousness being at the basis of the body, MAV offers more detail in its model of the mind/body as a dynamic pattern of intelligence. The next chapter discusses some more specific elements of the MAV model of physiology, which, together with the material already covered, provide the foundation for the daily practice of MAV.

REFERENCES

Faith R E, Murgo A J, Plotnikoff N P 1991 Interactions between the immune system and the nervous system. In: Plotnikoff N P et al Stress and immunity. CRC, Boca Raton, pp 287–303
Hillhouse J E, Kiecolt-Glaser J K, Glaser R 1991 Stress-associated modulation of the immune response in humans. In: Plotnikoff N P et al Stress and immunity. CRC, Boca Raton, pp 3–27
Maharishi Mahesh Yogi 1966 On the Bhagavad-Gita: a new translation and commentary, chapters 1–6. Penguin, London, p 128

5

Foundations of Ma...
Ayur-Veda's approac...
physiology and anato...

We said in Chapter 1 that standard medical training is unlikely to concern itself with defining 'health' as a positive concept. Its usual focus is disease, whose absence is called 'health' by default. Maharishi Ayur-Veda (MAV), by contrast, defines health and aims to create it actively.

How, then, does it define health? Sushruta, the author of one of the two major Ayurvedic texts (the other was Charaka) defined it this way: 'He whose *doshas* are in balance, whose appetite is good, whose *dhatus* are functioning normally, whose *malas* are in balance, and whose body, mind, and senses remain full of bliss, is called a healthy person' (*Sushruta*, Samhita, 15, 41). Clearly, Sushruta had something specific in mind when he talks about health; but equally clearly, a good deal of background is needed to understand what it is. What are *doshas*, *malas*, and *dhatus*?

In Chapter 2, we spoke about the core Ayurvedic concept of consciousness as the basis of the mind and body. This chapter will introduce some core elements of the MAV model of physiology and anatomy, beginning with an analysis of the fundamental principles called *doshas*, and going on to discuss the first expression of the *doshas* in the *dhatus*, the principles that uphold the formation of the bodily tissues. We will also examine the waste products of the *dhatus*, the *malas*, and the *shrotas*, or anatomical and physiological channels for the flow of biological information through the body, ranging from the most minute channels to the largest ones. Empirically, these concepts have proven very useful in understanding and treating difficult clinical symptoms and in individualizing treatments to suit the patient.

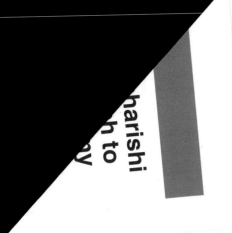

...gy differs from ...cine, some con- ...in approaching ...ologist Walter ... emerged from ... of the 19th century French physiologist Claude Bernard, who argued that 'all the vital mechanisms, varied as they are, have only one object, that of preserving constant the conditions of life in the internal environment'. The body can keep a relatively constant 'internal environment' through reference to thermostat-like setpoints. (We say 'relatively' constant, because the setpoints vary over the course of the day and year, as we discuss in a later chapter.) Body temperature is a familiar example, and the body has thousands of other homeostatic mechanisms, which regulate everything from blood oxygen levels to complex kidney functions that maintain fluid balances.

For thousands of years, Ayurveda has discussed an underlying, and at the same time overarching, sort of homeostasis – master homeostatic mechanisms that lie at the basis of all the other ones. Disruption of this overall internal balance, it holds, plays a basic role in the formation of *all* disease. While modern medicine focuses on destroying pathogenic invaders from outside the body, MAV focuses on making the body's defenses as strong as possible through promoting this inner balance. If this balance is maintained, immune strength is maximum, and degeneration is minimum. The person who does not catch the cold that is going around, MAV predicts, is the one whose physiology has maintained its inner balance better than those of the cold sufferers. And if we want to cure disease and later prevent its recurrence, a crucial element is restoring this overall balance.

The foundation of this overall balance is three organizing principles called the *doshas*. The ancient Ayurvedic texts discuss the *doshas* in what we would recognize as homeostatic terms. Disease can be caused by an excess of the *dosha*, or a shortage of the *dosha*. It can also be caused by 'vitiation' of the *dosha* – a dislodging of the *doshas* from their normal spheres of influence.

The exact nature of the *doshas* is discussed below. For now, let us note that in MAV the *doshas* are regarded as among the first sproutings of the unmanifest field of consciousness into the manifest realm of matter. If the *doshas* are balanced, MAV holds, the organizing power and balance at the basis of nature are infused into the more diversified material level of the body, and foster its healthy functioning. If the *doshas* are not balanced, the body has only partial access to nature's intelligence – a precondition for disease. All the procedures covered in this book, although they may also have more specific purposes, are designed to help establish balance in the three *doshas*.

As a first approximation, we might think of the three *doshas* in terms of broad functions. All natural systems, however else they differ, include at least three functions: motion, energy production, and structure. We might regard these as three categories into which all functions will fit. Our bodies, for example, have their *motion* systems: the impulses traveling through the nerves, the circulation of the blood, the progress of food through the digestive tract. They also have their *energy* component: the metabolic processes, the enzymes which digest the food and extract energy from it, and the cells' energy-producing chemical reactions. And finally, they have their solid physical *structure*: the bones, muscle, fat, and flesh. These three basic factors – motion, combustion, and structure – are not exact translations, but provide a good place to begin understanding the three *doshas*. *Vata* is the *dosha* which is expressed in all motion; *Pitta* is the one which is expressed in metabolism, heat production, digestion, and energy production; and *Kapha* gives solidity and structure, and balances the fluids.

To be more specific, *Vata* expresses itself as the activity of the locomotor system, and in functions such as blood circulation and the expansion and contraction of the lungs and heart. It also is involved in intestinal peristalsis and elimination, activities of the nervous system, the contractile process in muscle, ionic transport across membranes (such as the sodium pump), cell division, and unwinding of DNA during the process of transcription or replication. *Vata* is of prime importance in all homeostatic mechanisms.

Pitta (heat and metabolism) is exemplified by all metabolic activities, biochemical reactions, and the process of energy exchange. For example, it is concerned with digestion, functions of the exocrine glands and endocrine hormones, and intracellular metabolic pathways such as glycolysis, the tricarboxylic acid cycle, and the respiratory chain.

Kapha governs the structure and cohesion of the organism. It is responsible for biological strength, natural tissue resistance, and proper body structure. Microscopically, it is related to anatomical connections in the cell, such as the intracellular matrix, cell membrane, membranes of organelles, and synapses. On the level of biochemistry, it structures receptors and the various forms of chemical binding.

HOW THE *DOSHAS* INFLUENCE HEALTH

The three *doshas* are held to operate throughout nature. In an ecosystem, *Vata* is expressed in the wind, and the motion of water currents; sunshine is the most obvious example of *Pitta*, and fire another; and *Kapha* is expressed in the solid structures of the system – rocks, earth, etc. In nature, however, the *doshas* can seem to get out of balance. A hurricane can be thought of as an imbalance of *Vata*, a blazing heat wave an imbalance of *Pitta*, and a flood or blizzard an imbalance of *Kapha*. In the same way, our *doshas* can get imbalanced, and those imbalances are the basis of disease. For example, insomnia usually reflects an imbalance of *Vata*, the principle of movement, which when aggravated becomes overactive and creates too much mental activity at night; heartburn and ulcers result from imbalanced *Pitta*, the heat principle, which when aggravated 'burns' too much.

When they function normally, however, these same *doshas* produce the symptoms of good health. Because the *doshas* involve both the mind and the body, their effects are both mental and physical. Moreover, because the *doshas* are so basic, their range of effects is vast. Table 5.1 lists the characteristics that pertain when the *doshas* are balanced, and Table 5.2 some symptoms of imbalance and the *doshas* they relate to.

Vata as the 'lead' *dosha*

Because of its quality of mobility, *Vata* is said to 'lead' the other *doshas*. The other two *doshas* are considered

Table 5.1 Signs of balanced *doshas*

Vata	Pitta	Kapha
Exhilaration	Contentment Courage, dignity	Affection, generosity
Alertness	Sharp, clear intellect	Stability of mind
Normal formation of tissues	Normal heat and thirst mechanisms	Normal joints
Normal elimination	Good digestion	Muscular strength
Sound sleep	Lustrous complexion	Vitality

Table 5.2 Symptoms of imbalanced *doshas*

Vata	Pitta	Kapha
Dry or rough skin	Rashes, inflammatory skin diseases	Oily skin
Insomnia		Excessive sleep Lethargy, mental dullness
Constipation	Inflammatory bowel disease	Slow digestion
Common fatigue (non-specific causation)	Visual problems	Sinus congestion Nasal allergies
Tension headaches	Peptic ulcers, heartburn	Asthma
Intolerance of cold	Excessive body heat	
Degenerative arthritis	Premature graying or baldness	Cysts and other growths
Underweight		Obesity
Anxiety, worry	Hostility, irritability	

'lame'; they cannot move on their own. *Vata*, by contrast, is highly mobile and unstable, and thus prone to being aggravated. This results in one of the key ways that *doshas* cause disease: they become dislocated from their normal sites in the physiology (discussed in a later section). Aggravated *Vata* can lead to aggravation and dislocation of the other *doshas* – thus its role as leader or 'king' of the *doshas*. This is also why aggravation of *Vata* is much more likely to cause disease than aggravation of the other *doshas*; classical texts attribute about 80 types of disease to *Vata*, 40 to *Pitta*, and 20 to the highly stable *Kapha*.

How clinicians use the *dosha* concept

In treating any disease, the MAV doctor determines which *dosha* or combination of *doshas* is out of balance and takes steps to normalize it. This allows him or her not only to treat the symptom – nasal allergies, for example – but also to attend to its underlying cause, aggravated *Kapha* in this case. By attending to the root cause of disease, one can produce lasting improvements and strengthen the system as a whole. Moreover, it lets one take steps to prevent recurrences: for example, if we can keep *Kapha* balanced, the allergies will not return.

The three-*dosha* concept allows physicians to understand diseases that resist ordinary medical understanding, and to treat such diseases using natural means. Examples are chronic constipation, insomnia, and flatulence; by using the *dosha* theory, the physician can understand these diseases and, by attending to the underlying doshic imbalance that causes them, can treat them with an effectiveness that is often surprising.

PINNING DOWN THE *DOSHAS* MORE EXACTLY: THE *MAHABHUTAS* AND SPIN TYPES

Most MAV-trained physicians find the *dosha* concept to be useful in many ways. But many still have difficulty grasping exactly what the *doshas are*. We can understand elements of the body when they are *things* – we can imagine what a liver or a bone is like – but what is a '*dosha*'?

One way to look at the three *doshas* is simply as classification categories: all bodily functions can be fit into one of these categories, and this classification tells us a great deal about how to handle that function. This might be considered an example of thinking of the body as a dynamic pattern of knowledge. Another approach is found in Vedic theory. Again, these view the *doshas* as among the first manifestations of consciousness into the realm of matter, and as being formed from combinations of the five more basic 'elements' (*mahabhutas*) from which the entirety of creation is derived. The *mahabhutas* are held to be prior sproutings of consciousness into matter than *doshas*.

These five *mahabhutas* can, at first glance, appear to be remote from science, in that they are translated as 'space' (sometimes translated as 'ether'), air, fire, water, and earth; and according to classical Ayurveda, *Vata* derives from a combination of space and air, *Pitta* from fire and water, and *Kapha* from water and earth. But a more careful examination shows that this classification has remarkable correspondences with the modern physical theory we discussed in Chapter 2.

The physicist Dr John Hagelin, who has done important work in grand unification theory and is also the leading theorist on the parallels between Vedic Science and modern physics, told us a story from his graduate school days at Harvard. He was attending a seminar by a Nobel Laureate physicist, who quipped that the ancients had only five elements when now we know there are 92 chemical elements and dozens, if not hundreds, of more elementary particles. Hagelin responded by saying, 'I think physics is now back to five elements.' Having raised the group's collective eyebrow, Hagelin pointed out that quantum physics derives everything in creation from basic 'force' and 'matter' fields, and that all of these fields belong to one of five fundamental 'spin types'. These spin types are perhaps the most basic concept in particle physics; knowing them tells a physicist enormous amounts about the nature of particles. We could think of them as being like the primary colors, blue, red, and yellow: all the other colors of the rainbow are really combinations of these fundamental hues (orange, for example, is red plus yellow). In the same way, every possible material or force in the universe is a precipitate of the five spin types. They can, therefore, be described as the five true 'elements'.

Dr Hagelin forgot about the idea – it seemed an interesting curiosity – until years later, when he learned about Ayurveda and its five elements. He noted that each of the five spin types in physics corresponded very specifically to one of Ayurveda's five *mahabhutas* (elements). For example, the spin-2 'graviton', the highest spin type, which is responsible for curving space, corresponds to the highest *mahabhuta*, which happens also to be 'space' (*akasha*). The third in the series, the spin-1 force fields, includes electromagnetism, responsible for light, heat, and chemical transformations; it corresponds to the third *mahabhuta*, 'fire', which is responsible for the sense of sight (photons or light particles are spin-1 fields), for heat and for chemical transformations. The lowest spin type, Higgs Fields, is responsible for giving the other fields their mass; it corresponds to the lowest *mahabhuta*, the structure-giving 'earth'. The other spin types and *mahabhutas* corresponded as well (Table 5.3).

This still seemed just an interesting coincidence. What suggested to Hagelin that there may be a real connection between the ancient and the modern con-

Table 5.3 The five *mahabhutas* or "great elements" and the five spin types of modern physics

Five *mahabhutas*	Five spin types
Akasha (space)	Spin 2 = Graviton (gravity)
Vayu (air)	Spin $\frac{3}{2}$ = Gravitino
Tejas (fire)	Spin 1 = Force fields (electromagnetism)
Jala (water)	Spin $\frac{1}{2}$ = Matter fields
Prithivi (earth)	Spin 0 = Higgs fields

ceptions was noticing that the five spin types combine in three unexpected ways to give what are called the three 'superfields' – and that the five *mahabhutas* combine in exactly the same patterns to give the three *doshas*. Water and earth combine to form *Kapha*, while spin $\frac{1}{2}$ and spin 0, the corresponding spin types, combine to form the 'matter' superfield, which corresponds to *Kapha*. The combination that surprised Hagelin was *Pitta dosha*: the 'gauge' superfield, which has properties that correspond to *Pitta*, is formed of spins 1 and $\frac{1}{2}$, the equivalents of fire and water – but he had assumed that *Pitta* would be composed of fire and air. When he learned that traditionally *Pitta* is indeed held to be formed of fire and water, it seemed to him a corroboration of the possibility that physics and Ayurveda were using two different languages to describe the same reality (Fig. 5.1).

The mind and body have generally been thought of as macroscopic and thus not reflecting any medically significant quantum physical properties. It is possible that these and other correspondences between modern physics and MAV may help contribute to the development of a quantum mechanical understanding of the functioning of mind and body. If so, it would greatly

extend our understanding of health and how to achieve it. The analogy between superfields and *doshas*, should it prove to be more than an analogy, would certainly fit the traditional MAV concept of *doshas* as existing at a profound stratum of creation, rather than on the surface – as being among the first manifestations of the material world. In the meantime, what hundreds of Western doctors and thousands of patients are finding is that the *dosha/mahabhuta* theory works very effectively in clinical application.

In terms of their presence in the body, in fact, we can think of the *mahabhutas* as follows: *akasha* (space – in the body, channels); *vayu* (air – in the body gaseous exchange, O_2, CO_2, breathing); fire (chemical reactions, enzymatic activity, digestion); water (fluids, ionic constituents); and earth (solid structure).

THE QUALITIES OF THE *DOSHAS*

Traditional Ayurvedic texts associate each *dosha* with specific qualities, based on the elements that constitute the *dosha*. *Vata* is associated with 'cold, dryness, speed, and lightness'; *Pitta* with 'heat, sharpness, acidity'; *Kapha* with 'cold, heaviness, oiliness, and slowness'. These qualities are held to be subtle, rather than gross, tendencies: *Pitta* isn't thought of as a chemical, but as an essential principle, so 'heat and acidity' aren't meant to suggest that it is hot like sulfuric acid. The qualities of the *doshas* are more abstract. Still, the acid chemicals in the stomach which digest foods derive from *Pitta*. These qualities are used to categorize the effects of different treatments and regimens for balancing the *doshas*.

Principle of similars and opposites

The basic principle here is that similar (*samanya*) factors cause the increase or growth of the *dosha*, and opposite (*vishesha*) factors cause its decrease or diminution. *Vata*, for example, would be modulated by anything warm and moist – that is, anything with qualities opposite to *Vata* – while *Pitta* would be reduced by, among other things, cooling factors. For a *Vata* disease like lower back pain, one would use, among other treatments, wet heat on the back to reduce the cold, dry *Vata*; for a *Pitta* problem like

Akasha (space) and $\Rightarrow$ *Vata* *Vayu* (air)	Spin 2 and Spin $\frac{3}{2}$ $\Rightarrow$ Gravity	
Tejas (fire) and $\Rightarrow$ *Pitta* *Jala* (water)	Spin 1 and Spin $\frac{1}{2}$ $\Rightarrow$ Gauge	
Prithivi (earth) and $\Rightarrow$ *Kapha* *Jala* (water)	Spin 0 and Spin $\frac{1}{2}$ $\Rightarrow$ Matter	

Figure 5.1 The three *doshas* (as combinations of the five *mahabhutas*) and the three superfields (as combinations of the five spin types)

Table 5.4 Qualities of the *doshas* and their effects

Dosha	Qualities	Effects
Vata	1. Dry, rough (*rooksha*)	Dryness, emaciation, broken or hoarse voice, insomnia
	2. Light (*laghu*)	Light, inconsistent digestion, movement, and gait
	3. Mobile (*chala*)	Unstable, constantly moving joints, eyes, etc.
	4. Abundant (*bahu*)	Talkative; prominent tendons and veins
	5. Cold (*sheeta*)	Intolerant of cold; feels cold quickly
	6. Coarse, brittle (*khara*)	Rough, dry skin, rough hair
	7. Non-slimy (*vishada*)	Limbs and joints 'crack'
Pitta	1. Slightly oily (*sasneha*)	Smooth skin
	2. Hot, warm (*ushna*)	Intolerance for heat, excessive hunger, thirst; skin problems; early wrinkles, graying, and baldness
	3. Sharp (*teekshna*)	Physical strength, strong digestive power, sharpness
	4. Liquid (*drava*)	Loose, soft joints and muscles; tendency to sweat, more frequent urination than usual, tendency to looseness of bowel movements
	5. Sour (*amla*)	Fewer progeny, low sperm count
	6. Pungent (*katu*)	Fewer progeny, low sperm count
Kapha	1. Heavy (*guru*)	Stable gait; tendency to heavy build
	2. Cold (*sheeta*)	Slow, non-intense hunger, thirst, and perspiration
	3. Soft (*mrdhu*)	Pleasing appearance, milky, soft complexion
	4. Oily (*snigdha*)	Unctuous skin, organs
	5. Sweet (*madhura*)	Sweetness of speech and behavior
	6. Stable, steady (*sthira*)	Slow to anger, and to initiate actions

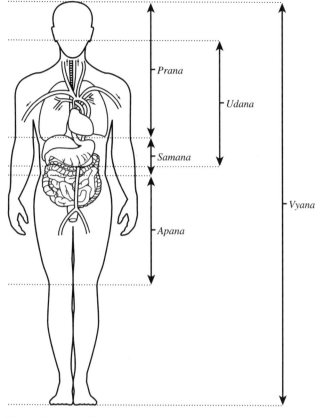

Figure 5.2 Locations of the five subdivisions of *Vata*

origin of a disease and the most important avenues of treatment. The following is a review of the subdivisions and locations of the *doshas*.

hyperacidity, one would avoid hot spicy foods and use other *Pitta*-reducing treatments.

Table 5.4 presents a more detailed list of the qualities of the *doshas* and the manifestation of these qualities in the mind and body.

THE FIVE *SUBDOSHAS*, AND THE *DOSHAS'* LOCATIONS

The functioning of the *doshas* is understood in terms more precise than those given above. Each *dosha* is said to have five subdivisions, and each of these is said to have natural locations in the body where its influence is especially evident. MAV physicians use this knowledge constantly in daily practice, and in locating the

The subdivisions of *Vata* (Fig. 5.2)

1. Prana vata

Location: The brain, head, throat, heart and respiratory organs.

Functions: *Prana vata* is responsible for respiration, which in itself makes it pre-eminently important. It is responsible for clarity of mind and reasoning, and supports memory and enthusiasm. It supports feeling, and governs perception through all the senses, especially hearing and touch. It is also responsible for such respiratory dysfunctions as sneezing and belching.

Conditions that result from imbalance: Respiratory disorders, cognitive problems, neurological disorders, tension headaches. Worry, anxiety, overly active mind, insomnia, hiccups, asthma. Just as *Vata*, is said to lead the other *doshas*, *prana vata* is said to lead the other *Vata doshas*. This makes it the most important *subdosha* to keep balanced.

2. Udana vata

Location: Navel, lungs, throat.

Function: *Udana vata* is responsible for the physiology of speech (and singing); it also relates to energy, ability to make an effort, strength, and also for the crucial act of swallowing.
Conditions that result from imbalance: Speech disorders; diseases of the throat (such as dry coughs and sore throats); fatigue.

3. Samana vata

Location: Stomach, intestines.

Function: 'Fans' the *Pitta* that digests food (discussed below); responsible for peristaltic motion.
Conditions that result from imbalance: Irregular or weak digestion, anorexia, bloating.

4. Apana vata

Location: Colon, bladder, navel, thighs, groin, sexual organs, rectum.

Function: Elimination of wastes. Sexual discharge, menstruation. The colon, the location of *apana vata*, is considered principal seat of *Vata*.
Conditions that result from imbalance: Constipation, diarrhea, flatulence, colitis, lower back pain and spasms, sexual dysfunctions, menstrual problems, genitourinary diseases.

5. Vyana vata

Location: Diffused throughout the body in the skin, nervous system, and circulatory system.

Function: Circulation, blood pressure, and the sense of touch.
Conditions that result from imbalance: Circulatory

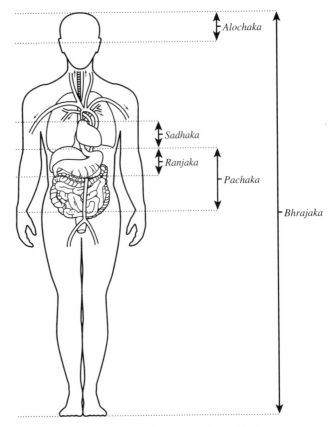

Figure 5.3   Locations of the five subdivisions of *Pitta*

and heart diseases, such as high blood pressure and heart arrhythmia. Nervous diseases. Often involved in other pathological processes.

The subdivisions of *Pitta* (Fig. 5.3)

1. Pachaka pitta

Location: Stomach and small intestines.

Function: Digestion of food, separation of waste products. Naturally, these are centrally important functions; as explained in the chapter on digestion, MAV regards them as even more central to disease and health than we are used to assuming.
Conditions that result from imbalance: Digestive weakness, heartburn, hyperacidity, ulcers.

2. Ranjaka pitta

Location: Liver, spleen, duodenum, red blood cells.

Function: The word '*ranjaka*' comes from the Sanskrit verb meaning 'to color'; it is responsible for the formation of red blood cells and otherwise balances the blood chemistry. It is aggravated by, among other things, toxins such as pollutants.

Conditions that result from imbalance: Anemia, blood disorders, jaundice, certain skin problems, anger and hostility (as in the ancient belief, preserved in such phrases as 'venting one's spleen').

3. Sadhaka pitta

Location: The heart.

Function: *Sadhaka pitta* is concerned especially with emotion, with contentment, and with memory and intelligence.

Conditions that result from imbalance: Depression and other psychiatric disturbances; heart disease; memory loss; indecisiveness.

4. Alochaka pitta

Location: Eyes

Function: Eyesight.

Conditions that result from imbalance: Visual problems in general; bloodshot eyes.

5. Bhrajaka pitta

Location: Skin.

Function: Skin metabolism.

Conditions that result from imbalance: Skin diseases, especially those of a *Pitta* nature such as boils, rashes, and acne.

The subdivisions of *Kapha* (Fig. 5.4)

1. Kledaka kapha

Location: Stomach.

Function: Moistening and initial digestion of food.

Conditions that result from imbalance: Dull digestion; imbalances of *kledaka* affect all the other *kaphas*.

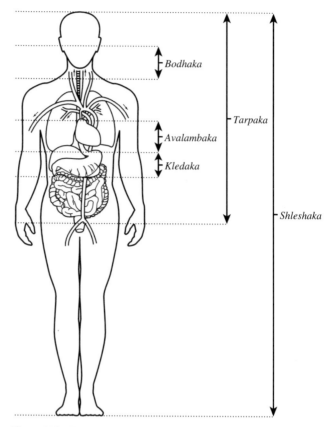

Figure 5.4 Locations of the five subdivisions of *Kapha*

2. Avalambaka kapha

Location: Chest, heart, lungs, and lumbar regions.

Function: Supports heart and lumbar region. Gives strength and stamina, especially in these regions and in upper torso.

Conditions that result from imbalance: Back pain, heart problems, chest congestion, asthma, wheezing, lethargy.

3. Bodhaka kapha

Location: Tongue, throat.

Function: Moistening the tongue, secretion of mucus in the mouth, and perception of taste. The last named is especially important in MAV (see Chapter 7).

Conditions that result from imbalance: Disruption of taste and salivation.

4. Tarpaka kapha

Location: The head, sinuses, and cerebrospinal fluid.

Function: Moistening the nose, mouth, and eyes; maintaining spinal fluid; nourishment of the mind and of the sense and motor organs.

Conditions that result from imbalance: Sinus problems, nasal congestion, cough coming from upper respiratory tract, sinus headaches, problems with the senses, especially of smell.

5. Shleshaka kapha

Location: Joints.

Function: Lubrication of joints throughout the body. Cohesion and binding all over the body.

Conditions that result from imbalance: Joint problems.

THE *DOSHAS* AND PATHOGENESIS

Since MAV views all disease as resulting from disruption of the natural balance of the *doshas*, it follows that the *doshas* play a key role in its approach to understanding pathogenesis. In Western medicine, a disease is usually detected as a result of its symptoms. Unfortunately, in most diseases, the symptoms emerge fairly late in the process of pathogenesis. Obviously, the earlier in the process we could detect the disease, the better chance we would have of controlling and curing it.

As we will see in detail in Chapter 6, MAV locates six stages of pathogenesis, the first three of which have highly subtle symptoms with which allopathic medicine is not familiar. These first three stages involve aggravation of the normal functioning of the *doshas*. The later stages have the *dosha* wandering to and then localizing in an unsuitable location, where it disrupts health. A skilled MAV diagnostician can detect the early pathogenic stages before overt symptoms emerge, using diagnostic techniques discussed later in the book, such as Ayurvedic examination of the pulse. It is especially helpful in preventive medicine.

Below we examine a more basic principle: people who have a predominance of one of the *doshas* are more likely to develop ailments related to that *dosha*.

SUMMARY: THE *DOSHAS*

We have stated that the MAV model sees the body as a dynamic pattern of knowledge; here we see one way in which that idea is applied. The *dosha* concept deals with the body at a more abstract level than is usual in medicine: it concerns us not just with organ systems or even cells or molecules, but with more abstract underlying patterns. We have speculated that these may have some connection to the abstract patterns found in physics.

The three-*dosha* theory may someday prove valuable in scientific understanding of, for example, typology (see next section). But its main value is clinical. Using the *doshas* allows one to customize treatment to the individual with great specificity, to come up with an effective general approach to prevention, and much else. This becomes obvious when one begins to make use of the MAV concept of *dosha* predominance.

PREDOMINANT *DOSHAS*

BALANCING THE *DOSHAS*

One Ayurvedic phrase that often needs clarification is 'to balance the *doshas*'. Imbalances in the *doshas* create the ground for disease, and balance of the *doshas* creates health. But the term 'balance' can mislead us into thinking that the doctor attempts to produce equal amounts of each *dosha*. In fact, while everyone has all three *doshas* – everyone needs solid structure (*Kapha*), energy (*Pitta*), and motion (*Vata*) in their body – the appropriate relative amounts differ in different people. 'Balancing the *doshas*' has nothing to do with amounts, but rather with fostering the normal, healthy functioning of each *dosha*.

The differing proportions of *doshas* give rise to different predominant functional *doshas*. These types are especially central to MAV treatment. The first question a MAV physician asks is not 'What disease does my patient have?' but 'What predominant functional *doshas* does my patient have?' This is because different predominances are susceptible to different diseases and respond differently to different treatments. Side-effects are much more easily avoided if you know the patient's predominant *doshas*, and the correct treatment program for a specific patient becomes much more apparent.

The most obvious principles of *dosha* predominance can be easily grasped. The *doshas* have distinctive characteristics, and they impart a particular style or tone to everyone's psychophysiology. If you go to get a new driver's license and watch people trapped in a long line, you can get some idea of their underlying doshic make-up. People who appear anxious and worried – who fidget, look over their shoulder, look at their watch, wring their hands – are likely to be *Vata* predominants. People who look red-faced and angry, who glare piercingly around, push for position, and yell at the clerks – are likely to be predominantly *Pitta*. People who seem content and at ease – who may look plump or stolid, and who sit patiently without so much as picking up something to read – are likely to be predominantly *Kapha*.

We now consider the three 'main' forms of doshic predominance in more detail and then look at how physicians can use that knowledge to create better health (Table 5.5).

VATA PREDOMINANTS
Physical characteristics

People whose constitutions are dominated by *Vata* tend to be thin, with smaller frames. *Vatas*' joints tend to 'crack' noisily, and may be protuberant. *Vatas* become cold easily, especially in wintertime. Their eyes tend to be smaller and their hair may be curly or kinky. They have dry skin.

They need less sleep than other types – 6 hours is usually sufficient – but may have more trouble getting it, for their sleep tends to be light. Because they are easily awakened, their night of sleep may be interrupted by periods of wakefulness. They tend to be very active, but may overdo it and become fatigued or exhausted. This can lead to generalized feelings of physical weakness or fatigue, especially if their sleep is troubled.

Vata appetites are irregular, sometimes strong and sometimes weak. *Vatas* tend towards constipation.

Cognitive characteristics

Vata predominants tend to be very alert, with quick,

Table 5.5 The three main *dosha* predominances

Vata	Pitta	Kapha
Light, thin build	Moderate build	Solid, heavier build
Acts quickly	Acts with medium speed	Slow, methodical
Averse to cold weather	Averse to hot weather	Averse to damp weather
Irregular digestive power, irregular appetite	Strong digestion, sharp appetite	Slow digestion, mild appetite
Quick to learn	Medium time to learn	Slow to learn
Quick to forget	Medium memory	Slow to forget
Tendency to worry	Tends to anger	Tranquil, steady
Tendency to constipation	Regular elimination sometimes loose or frequent stools	Regular elimination
Vivacious, always moving		
Light, interrupted sleep, about 6 hours	Sound sleep, medium length	Heavy, long sleep
Tends to fatigue, less physical stamina	Enterprising, sharp	Stamina, strength
Curly hair more likely	Thin, fair hair	Dark, full hair
Dry skin	Reddish complexion, moles and freckles	Oily, smooth skin
Prominent joints, tendons, and veins	Early graying or balding	

active minds. They grasp new concepts and learn new things quickly. They have excellent short-term memories, but may not remember things well over the long term: they are quick to learn and quick to forget.

Psychological characteristics

Vatas tend to move, think, and speak quickly. If *Vata dosha* is balanced, they are creative and enthusiastic. They make friends quickly and have many acquaintances. If *Vata dosha* is out of balance, though, they tend to blame themselves, to worry, be anxious, be overly sensitive, and have difficulty making decisions.

PITTA PREDOMINANTS
Physical characteristics

Pittas tend towards moderate height and body frames. Their complexion is generally fair or reddish or copper-like. They have thin and silky hair which is often red, blond, or light brown. Premature graying or baldness is a symptom of a *Pitta* constitution, as are moles and freckles.

Pitta predominants generally have strong digestion and strong appetites. Missing a meal or getting it late can be an ordeal for them, as the delay may make them fatigued or irritable. Their elimination may be regular, or it may tend towards frequent or loose bowel movements. Their sleep at night is sound and of medium length.

Because *Pitta* is warm by nature, *Pitta* predominants tend to be averse to hot weather and to prolonged exposure to the sun. They perspire and get overheated more than other types. They prefer cold food and drinks.

Cognitive characteristics

Pittas tend to have sharp, penetrating intellects. Their minds are methodical and well-organized.

Psychological characteristics

When *Pitta* is balanced, *Pitta* predominants can be bold, courageous, focused, organized, perceptive, energetic, and chivalrous. Enterprising by nature, they make excellent leaders – bosses are often *Pitta* predominant. They tend to be very good public speakers. They enjoy competition and prefer competitive sports. When *Pitta* is out of balance, though, the *Pitta* predominant may speak harshly or critically. They may be stubborn and overly perfectionistic. Preferring an orderly environment, they will impose order on a disorganized one. When balanced, *Pittas* can be sweet, but when out of balance, they can be short-tempered, impatient, and sharp in dealing with others.

KAPHA PREDOMINANTS
Physical characteristics

Kapha is responsible for giving substance to the body, and the *Kapha*-dominated constitution tends to be well-developed and rounded, with a broad chest and good musculature. *Kaphas* gain weight easily, however, and may tend towards obesity. Their skin is usually soft, lustrous, and oily, and their complexion light or fair. Thick, dark, soft, and wavy hair is a *Kapha* characteristic, and *Kaphas* also tend to have large, soft eyes with long eyelashes, and strong white teeth.

Their digestion tends to be slow, and they may feel heavy after meals. Usually they have a mild appetite, and they easily tolerate missing a meal. The bowel patterns of *Kapha* predominants are very regular.

Kaphas have excellent physical stamina, but they need more sleep than other types to avoid feeling fatigued. Their sleep tends to be heavy and deep. They do not perspire much, and they dislike cool, damp weather.

Cognitive characteristics

Kaphas are 'slow to learn and slow to forget'. They may have to hear new information several times before they completely grasp it, but, once they do, they remember it for a long time.

Psychological characteristics

Kapha predominants tend to be tranquil and steady; they do not worry or get angry easily. Slow and calm in their activity, they are agreeable, forgiving, affectionate, generous, and emotionally stable. Their speech is clear, concise and unhurried. When *Kapha* is out of balance, though, they can be lethargic, overly attached to the status quo, and lacking in motivation.

MIXED INFLUENCES

An important qualification to the above: Most people are not purely *Vata*, *Pitta*, or *Kapha*. While everyone's body has a predominance of one or two *doshas*, it is usually a mixture such as *Kapha/Pitta*. Although we can understand the mixtures simply by combining the above three descriptions, MAV does locate some characteristics specific to each of them.

Vata/Pittas or *Pitta/Vatas*

Vata/Pittas or *Pitta/Vatas* are similar in build to the pure *Vata*, though if they have enough *Pitta* they may be stronger and more muscular than more sinewy *Vatas*. Like their *Vata* counterparts, they are quick-moving, friendly, and talkative, but they tend to be more enterprising and to have more sharp, focused intellects, and more energy, stamina and assertiveness. The addition of *Pitta* to the constitution gives greater stability and stronger digestion and more regular elimination. The *Vata/Pitta* also tolerates the cold better than pure *Vatas* do. In general, the pure *Vata* is highly sensitive to the environment, while the *Vata/Pitta* is less so. They tackle problems enthusiastically.

Pitta/Kaphas or *Kapha/Pittas*

Pitta/Kaphas and *Kapha/Pittas* combine the aggressiveness and sharp intellect of *Pitta* with the solid stability of *Kapha*. They are more muscular than the *Pitta/Vata* predominants, solid and sturdy rather than wiry or lean. A larger ratio of *Kapha* may give them a more rounded appearance, with a higher fat to muscle ratio. This is a particularly good constitution for athletes, because *Pitta* gives energy and fire while *Kapha* gives stamina, although a larger ratio of *Kapha* may reduce the inclination to exercise. *Pitta/Kaphas* may find it uncomfortable to miss a meal.

Vata/Kaphas

Vata/Kaphas have a thin and wiry build, though not to the extreme of the pure *Vata* predominant constitution. But their temperament differs markedly from the *Vata*. While *Vatas* are always in motion, the *Vata/Kapha* is more even-tempered, projecting a sense of inner stability and strength. Extra *Kapha* may make them more slow-moving. The *Vata/Kapha* is quick and efficient when action is called for, but otherwise has a calm and relaxed manner – 'coolheaded', reflecting the predominance of the cold *doshas*. Because of this predominance, their digestion may be irregular or slow, and they may be intolerant of the cold.

Vata/Pitta/Kaphas

Vata/Pitta/Kaphas (also called *samadoshas*) integrate the characteristics of the *Vata*, *Pitta*, and *Kapha* predominants. When such individuals balance their *doshas*, they enjoy the best qualities of the three pure types. Once those with *samadosha* are brought into balance, they are less likely to become imbalanced than are others, because the almost perfect equality of the *doshas* gives them tremendous stability and flexibility.

Each of these conditions has unique advantages and challenges. When balanced, each exhibits its best characteristics.

THE TWO TYPES OF *PRAKRITI* (PREDOMINANT *DOSHAS* IN PHYSIOLOGY) AND THE *VIKRITI* (CURRENT IMBALANCE IN *DOSHAS*)

Ayurvedic physicians refer to three kinds of predominant *doshas*. One is that found at birth, or the *janma prakriti*; a second is that found currently in the individual, or the *deha prakriti*; and the third is the current imbalances of the *doshas*, or *vikriti*. The *janma prakriti* is determined at conception, based on a number of factors, heredity being the most important. The *prakriti* may change slowly and gradually over the course of life as a result of a huge variety of factors, yielding the current *deha prakriti*.

The current doshic imbalances or *vikriti* can change rapidly. The *vikriti* results from impurities and imbalances which accumulate over the seasons and years. These imbalances, which can result from diet, lifestyle, stress, etc., interact with the *prakriti* to produce the *vikriti*. The *vikriti* often masks the *prakriti*.

Suppose one is predominantly a *Kapha* by *deha prakriti*, but that one's *Vata dosha* is severely imbalanced. One may *appear* to be *Vata* predominant. After Ayurvedic treatment, this person's physiology may be more balanced, and the true kaphic qualities will emerge. Worry and indecisiveness (which are symptoms of *imbalanced Vata*) had seemed part of their basic personality, but now turn out not to be.

Regular use of MAV over the years is said to remove imbalances in the physiology, so eventually the physician becomes increasingly certain of what the underlying *deha prakriti* is. Before then, what physicians commonly evaluate is the *vikriti*, the current state of imbalance.

WHAT IS MEANT BY BALANCING THE *DOSHAS*?

Now that we have a sense of *dosha* predominances

(*prakriti*) and imbalances (*vikriti*) we can discuss how 'balancing' the *doshas* can be of significant value for a clinician. The principle used is that people with a predominance of a certain *dosha* are more likely to develop diseases related to that *dosha*. Because the *dosha* is present in such abundance, even a fairly small increase or vitiation is more likely to cause illness. This helps determine effective preventive procedures. *Vata* predominants are more likely to ward off disease by taking steps (using diet, routine, etc.) to keep *Vata* in a state of balance, especially in *Vata*-aggravating seasons and situations; *Pittas* and *Kaphas* would apply the same principle to their respective *doshas*.

In later chapters, we will examine the means through which physician and patient can bring the *doshas* into their natural state of balance. These are, of course, crucial to MAV's approach to preventive medicine. All these approaches have to be customized to suit the individual's *Prakriti* and *Vikriti*.

OTHER ASPECTS OF MAV ANATOMY AND PHYSIOLOGY: THE *DHATUS*, *OJAS*, *MALAS*, AND *SHROTAS*

THE *DHATUS*

Another central element of Ayurvedic theory and practice involves what are known as the seven *dhatus*. The term is often translated as 'tissue elements', but is better understood as fundamental principles that support the various bodily tissues. The *dhatus* once again foreshadow the concept of homeostasis. The *Charaka Samhita*, section *Sutrasthana*, states: 'The very object of [Ayurveda] is the maintenance of the equilibrium of the *dhatus*' (I. 53). Charaka defines disease as 'any disturbance in the equilibrium of *dhatus*' and health as 'the state of their equilibrium' (IX. 4). Charaka also sees a homeostatic tendency *within* the *dhatus*: he says they 'come to normalcy irrespective of any external causative factors' (XVI. 27). The *dhatus* are disturbed, however, by various external factors, such as 'wrong utilization, non-utilization, and excessive utilization of time, mental faculties, and objects of the sense organs' (I. 54) – behavioral factors that are discussed in later chapters.

The seven *dhatus* are:

1. *Rasa dhatu* (the principle upholding the first products of digested food, such as chyle).
2. *Rakta dhatu* (the principle upholding blood).
3. *Mamsa dhatu* (the principle upholding muscle).
4. *Meda dhatu* (the principle upholding adipose tissue).
5. *Asthi dhatu* (the principle upholding bone).
6. *Majja dhatu* (the principle upholding bone marrow and nervous system).
7. *Shukra dhatu* (the principle upholding semen and sperm in males and ovum in females).

The *dhatus* are central to Ayurvedic diagnosis and treatment. For one thing, they can be used, like the *doshas*, in classifying the patient's *prakriti*. For another, again like the *doshas*, the seven *dhatus* are each said to give rise to certain symptoms and diseases when vitiated, and to give rise to certain positive health elements when balanced. Finally, certain factors are understood to vitiate specific *dhatus*, and other ones to balance specific *dhatus*. Below we examine each of these areas in turn.

Predominance of *dhatus*

Individual differences in the development of the *dhatus* are known as *sāras* or 'essences'. These refer not so much to the amount of the *dhatu* present as to the 'excellence' of the *dhatu*'s development and functioning. This might be used to further refine the information gained from looking at doshic predominance. A *Kapha* with a ruddy complexion may, for example, also have very healthy, well-developed *rakta*. The excellent development of a particular *dhatu* might produce various obvious signs; some examples are as follows:

- *Rasa*: unctuous and smooth, soft, lustrous skin; clear, fine, deep-rooted hair.
- *Rakta*: unctuous and ruddy face.
- *Mamsa*: stable, large, well-formed musculature.
- *Meda*: oily complexion; healthy plumpness (not obesity).
- *Asthi*: well-formed bones and joints.
- *Majja*: softness of organs; long, rounded joints.
- *Shukra*: gentle look, milky whites of eyes, clear and unctuous complexion.

Vitiation of *dhatus*

For diseases arising from *dhatu* vitiation, the *dhatus* might be considered along with the *doshas* in analyzing a disease. Hypertension, for example, involves the *subdoshas vyana* and *prana vata*, and *sadhaka* and *tarpaka pitta*; but it also involves *rasa* and *rakta dhatus*.

The longest list of diseases related to *dhatus* are those based on *rasa* (the products of digestion), and *rakta* (blood); this is not surprising, since these *dhatus* precede the genesis of all the other *dhatus*. Vitiation of *rasa* (the *dhatu* involving the digestive products of food) is said to give rise to such food-related disorders as anorexia, nausea, excessive leanness, foul taste in the mouth, loss of taste sensation, and loss of digestive power. It also can contribute to problems of vitality, such as heaviness, drowsiness, malaise, and impotence. In addition, it is held to contribute to untimely wrinkles and gray hair, leanness, body aches, paleness, and certain fevers.

Vitiation of *rakta*, the *dhatu* upholding blood, can give rise to erysipelas, boils, internal hemorrhaging, menorrhagia, spleen disorders, pustules, abscess, leukoderma, and various skin disorders. Vitiation of *mamsa* (muscle) involves cervical adenitis, keloids, tonsillar hypertrophy, skin disorders, and muscular wasting. Vitiation of *meda* (fat) can give rise to obesity, diabetes, excessive leanness, and hyperlipidemia. Vitiation of *asthi* (bone) involves abnormalities of hair, nails, beard, and teeth, as well as bone pain. Vitiation of *majja* (marrow) can give rise to dizziness, fainting, darkness of vision, and pain in the joints. Vitiation of *shukra* can give rise to impotence, infertility, and miscarriage.

Factors that disrupt (vitiate) the *dhatus*

The next MAV concern is with avoiding factors that disrupt the *dhatu's* balance. These are specific to each *dhatu*. *Rasa*, the *dhatu* concerned with the first products of digestion, is vitiated by overeating, especially when it involves cold, heavy or oily foods, which are harder to digest. Too much mental work can disrupt *rasa* too. *Rakta* is vitiated by too much exposure to heat and the sun, and overly hot foods and drinks. *Mamsa dhatu* is vitiated by overly heavy or bulky food, or foods that clog the *shrotas* (discussed below); *meda* is aggravated by lack of exercise, sleeping too much in the day, fatty

food, and alcohol; *asthi dhatu* by overexercise, excessive jerking movements, and constant use of *Vata*-aggravating food and behavior; and *majja* by crushing injuries, and certain toxic substances.

Vitiation of *shukra dhatu* (the reproductive fluids) can cause infertility. One of the things that vitiates *shukra* is excessive sexual indulgence. This might seem surprising, but is in tune with the understanding of modern andrology that abstinence is one of the most effective means of increasing sperm count. In strengthening *shukra* to increase fertility, such moderation might complement the use of foods and herbs (such as milk, ghee, urad dahl, and saffron) that strengthen *shukra*.

Ojas and the *dhatus*

The most important way to strengthen the *dhatus* is to increase the quantity of the biochemical called *ojas*, from which all the *dhatus* are said to arise. *Ojas* is in fact said to be the 'essence of the *dhatus*'. *Ojas* is also said to pervade the body. According to Charaka, when the quantity of *ojas* diminishes too much, life itself is threatened. Maharishi describes *ojas* as connecting consciousness and matter: *ojas*, he says, is like a lamp at the door, shining both inside and outside. Increasing *ojas*, therefore, helps increase the expression of awakened pure consciousness in individual life.

According to Ayurvedic theory, the seven *dhatus develop* in the sequence given above. The first *dhatu*, *rasa* (the principle upholding the first products of digestion) is metabolized by a specific 'digestive fire' or *agni*, and turned into the essence of the next *dhatu* (in this case, *rakta*, the principle upholding blood). In between one *dhatu* and the next, a specific type of *ojas* is formed, out of which the next *dhatu* is created. The type of *ojas* formed is different in each one of these stages; this yields, of course, eight types of *ojas* (Fig. 5.5).

The *dhatus* and the 13 *agnis*

The transformation of one *dhatu* to another is said to be metabolized by principles of transformation called *agnis*. The main *agni*, and first step in the digestive process, is the *jathar agni*, or digestive fire, which metabolizes food and supports all the other *agnis*; we

$$ojas \rightarrow rasi \Rightarrow rakta \Rightarrow mamsa \Rightarrow meda \Rightarrow ashti \Rightarrow majja \Rightarrow shukra \rightarrow ojas$$

$$\downarrow \qquad \downarrow \qquad \downarrow \qquad \downarrow \qquad \downarrow \qquad \downarrow$$

(ojas) (ojas) (ojas) (ojas) (ojas) (ojas)

Figure 5.5   The sequential development of the *dhatus*

Food (*ahara*)
↓ Gross digestion by the *jatharagni* (digestive fire in stomach and intestines)
↓

Ahara rasa
↓ Intermediate digestion by the five *bhutagnis*:

Akasha	Vayu	Tejas	Jala	Prithivi
agni	agni	agni	agni	agni

↓

20 *gunas* (qualities) of food
↓ Tissue metabolism by the seven *dhatu agnis*:

  Rasagni – Raktagni – Mamsagni – Medagni – Asthagni – Majjagni – Shukragni
↓
The seven *dhatus*

Figure 5.6   The digestive process and the 13 *agnis*

will talk about it more in our chapter on digestion. The next step in the digestive process involves the five *bhuta agnis*, which metabolize the five *mahabhutas*, and are called *akasha agni, vayu agni, tejas agni, jala agni,* and *prithivi agni*. The *bhuta agnis* are concerned with transformation on all levels of the physiology. The qualities of the *mahabhutas* that exist in food are transformed or metabolized by the *bhuta agnis*.

But the *agnis* that relate to our current focus, the seven *dhatus*, are called the seven *dhatu agnis* (*rasa agni, rakta agni,* and so forth) and metabolize the formation of each of the *dhatus* from the previous one and from *ojas* (Fig. 5.6).

THE *MALAS*

The *malas* are the body's waste products. They are formed as a by-product of the work of the *agnis* in metabolizing and transforming food and the *dhatus*. The principal *malas* are said to be urine (*mootra*), stool (*purisha*), and sweat (*sweda*); others include mucus, ear wax, nails, and so on.

The *malas* are of considerable importance in Ayurveda. The urine and stool, for example, are said to remove not only waste products of food, but also waste products of cellular metabolism, including unhealthful ones. Sweat also can have this function. We will discuss the idea of elimination of impurities in greater detail in the chapter on *panchakarma* (Ch. 10).

For now, let us note that although the *malas* contain all five *mahabhutas*, each is especially related to a specific *dhatu*. Mucus is said to be the waste product of *rasa* (chyle), and to be associated with *Kapha dosha*; bile is said to be the waste product of *rakta* (blood), and to be associated with *Pitta dosha*; the *khamalas* – excreta from outer orifices – are said to be associated with *mamsa* (muscle); sweat (*sweda*) is associated with *meda* (fat); hair is said to be the waste product of *asthi* (bone). Feces and urine are, of course, the waste products of food (*anna*).

THE *SHROTAS*

The *dhatus* are said to move and be transformed through subtle channels of circulation called *shrotas*, of which there are 13 types (see Table 5.6). The *shrotas* also convey the *malas*.

The *shrotas'* obstruction or vitiation is considered a crucial element in the etiology of disease. An obvious example of this in Western medicine is atherosclerosis, the thickening of blood vessel walls (*rakta vaha shrotas*) that leads to stiffness, brittleness, and narrowing of the passageway. This restricts the flow of blood to the cells, causing a wide range of damage – not just dramatic results like strokes, but slow losses, like decreased perfusion of blood to endocrine glands and resultant hormone depletion. Another type of *shrota* vitiation involves *excessive* flow (e.g. in dysentery). A third type

Table 5.6   The *shrotas*

Shrota	Its 'root' (*moola*) organ	What it carries
1. *Prana vaha shrotas*	Respiratory tract	Oxygen, 'vital force'
2. *Udaka vaha shrotas*	Palate, pancreas	Water, fluids
3. *Anna vaha shrotas*	Stomach	Food
4. *Rasa vaha shrotas*	Heart	Chyle, lymph, plasma
5. *Rakta vaha shrotas*	Liver, spleen	Blood
6. *Mamsa vaha shrotas*	Tendons, ligaments, skin	Ingredients of muscle tissue
7. *Meda vaha shrotas*	Kidneys, omentum	Ingredients of fat tissue
8. *Asthi vaha shrotas*	Hip bone	Ingredients of bone tissue
9. *Majja vaha shrotas*	Bones, joints	Ingredients of bone
10. *Shukra vaha shrotas*	Testes, ovaries	Semen, ovum
11. *Mootra vaha shrotas*	Kidneys, bladder	Urine
12. *Varco vaha shrotas*	Colon, rectum	Feces
13. *Sweda vaha shrotas*	Fat tissues, glands, skin	Sweat

involves *diverted* flow – such as improper shunting of the blood – and a fourth type structural changes – for example, the atheroma that develops in atherosclerosis.

Vitiation of the *shrotas* leads to vitiation of the *dhatus*, and vice versa. Both can be vitiated by the three *doshas*, or by food or regimens that aggravate the *doshas* or *dhatus*. Some examples of factors that vitiate the *shrotas* are overeating, eating before the previous meal is digested, unwholesome foods or those incompatible with each other (such as salt and milk, sour fruit and milk, or fish and milk), overexercise, too little exercise, excessive heat or cold, excessive worry, and concussion or shock.

SUMMARY: FOUNDATIONS OF MAV PRACTICE

Sushruta's definition of health – *doshas* in balance, good appetite (i.e. healthy *agnis*), normally functioning *dhatus*, balanced *malas* – involves four core ideas of Maharishi Ayur-Veda anatomy and physiology: the 3 *doshas*, the 13 *agnis*, the 7 *dhatus*, and the *malas*. This chapter introduced these ideas, along with some further concepts: the 15 *subdoshas*, the constitutional types based on *doshas*, the *shrotas*, and *ojas*. Together with the central idea of consciousness, discussed in Chapters 2, 3, and 4 (wherein lay another element of Sushruta's definition – the body, mind and senses being full of 'bliss'), these concepts provide a foundation for the rest of the book, which will refer to them in many different ways.

Chapters 2 through 4 dealt with more immaterial, more unmanifest realms of human existence: consciousness and the mind. This chapter considered the more manifest material realms, from its first sproutings in the *mahabhutas*, through its expression in the *doshas*, *dhatus*, and finally the *malas*. As will become evident in future chapters, which discuss such areas as diet and daily routine, almost any medical advice in MAV involves the balance or imbalance of *doshas*, *ojas*, and the *dhatus* in critical ways, and also is concerned with the more basic realm of the mind and, beneath it, consciousness.

6

Pathogenesis and diagnosis

What causes a patient to get sick? Western medicine has made enormous progress in uncovering immediate causes: a microbe, a toxin, a gene. But perhaps it is not enough for us to stop at this level of causation. Many people who are exposed to a microbe catch the cold or flu it causes, but others exposed to the same microbe remain healthy. Most people exposed to a carcinogen don't develop cancer. Some who develop cancers recover. Some who have HIV never develop AIDS. Understanding why a pathogen *does not* make some people sick is the next frontier in the war against disease.

It is precisely this frontier that Ayurvedic etiology has always occupied. Ancient Ayurvedic texts and tradition concerned themselves with factors of behavior, diet, and thought and feeling that make one *susceptible* to disease. In recent years, Western medicine has begun to examine all three areas, but it has much to learn from the Maharishi Ayur-Veda (MAV) approach. If we think of disease as unwanted weeds, Western medicine has focused on identifying and fighting the weeds through using, by analogy, herbicides; MAV has focused on keeping the grounds inhospitable to weeds, so that they cannot take root or flourish. When you remember that the seeds of disease – pathogens – are always present in abundance, and that microbes develop resistances to the chemicals we use to fight them, the MAV approach begins to seem timely and sensible.

Ayurvedic tradition locates *one ultimate cause of disease*, one underlying reason why the ground becomes especially hospitable to weeds: *pragya-aparadh*, the 'mistake of the intellect' discussed in Chapter 2. The very first step in the development of disease, MAV says, is a change in awareness deep inside. The first step in treatment should ideally be a change in the same area. Again, 'intellect' does not mean the faculty measured by IQ tests, but, rather, the basis of our discriminating between ourselves and everything else. The 'mistake' made at this level results in our being cut off from our own innermost nature. The intellect, becoming enamored of the material manifestations of consciousness, forgets its source in the underlying unity. One begins to choose in terms of the senses rather than the totality of life, and chooses unhealthy patterns of thought and behavior. Thus *pragya-aparadh* results in mistakes regarding behavior, diet (Ch. 7), daily and seasonal routine (Ch. 9), and so forth.

Pragya-aparadh has two subsidiary manifestations that also can be considered ultimate causes of disease:

1. *Asatmyaendriyartha samyoga*: unwholesome contact between sense organs and their objects. This presages current attempts to understand the influence of emotion on health. For example, to consider the sense of hearing, such contact might involve harsh, unwelcome, or emotionally disturbing words, as well as overly loud sounds (such as those that might cause deafness or tinnitus). Regarding the sense of sight this might involve staring at the sun, or living in too much winter darkness (for those with seasonal affective disorder syndrome), but also seeing emotionally upsetting or shocking sights (this may add a new, psychophysiological element to current debates about the effects of TV and movies on children and adults). Similar ideas are applied to the other organs of action and perception.
2. *Kala parinama*, which refers to the influence of time; this relates to the daily and seasonal routines we speak of in Chapter 9, and also to unseasonal weather conditions, such as snow in June in the northern hemisphere.

The three types of 'mistakes'

These most basic causes of disease create their effect by inducing *mistakes* in three areas: (1) diet, (2) regimen, and (3) mental activity. Each of these areas is discussed in chapters on diet, daily and seasonal routine, and behavioral *rasayanas*.

The three types of 'abnormalities'

Finally, these three kinds of mistakes lead to three types of *abnormalities*:

1. The *doshas* becoming out of balance (Ch. 5).
2. The *agnis* or digestive fires becoming weak or dull, and thus producing harmful *ama* instead of *ojas* as the end-products of digestion (Chs 4 and 5).
3. The *shrotas* (channels of circulation) becoming vitiated or clogged (Ch. 5).

For an example of a 'mistake' causing an 'abnormality', a mistake in regimen – exercising strenuously or straining mentally too late at night – could aggravate *prana vata*, and thus cause insomnia. A mistake in diet – eating a large amount of cold, heavy food late at night – could overburden the digestive fire (*jathar agni*), which results in *shrota*-clogging *ama*. A mistake in mental activity – indulging in jealous anger and backbiting – could contribute to cardiovascular and digestive disease.

The three types of abnormality are the principal causes of pathology in MAV clinical practice. To look at the causes of these three abnormalities in more detail:

1. Factors that aggravate the *doshas* include diet unsuited to the *doshas* that are predominant in that individual, daily and seasonal routines, exercise programs, and mental or behavioral tendencies that aggravate the *doshas*.
2. Factors that weaken the *agni* include overeating and, at the other extreme, fasting, as well as eating before the previous meal is digested, irregular eating, eating during indigestion, unwholesome food, eating food unsuitable to the season and individual, and eating when under the sway of emotions like anger and grief.
3. Factors that vitiate the *shrotas* are in some cases the same as those that vitiate the *agni* – overeating, eating before the previous meal is digested, eating unwholesome or incompatible foods – and in other cases quite different: too much or too little exercise, excessive heat or cold (and rapid alternation from one of these to the other), a concussion or shock, and excessive worry.

To summarize the causes of pathogenesis: mistakes in diet, regimen, or thinking lead to abnormalities in the *doshas*, *agni*, and *shrotas*. These abnormalities create the fertile ground in which disease takes root and flourishes. In treating a disease, the main thing a practitioner does is to try to remove these abnormalities.

Handling the cause

A key point here is that MAV attempts not only to treat the symptoms of disease but to locate and remove the cause (known as the *hetu* in classic Sanskrit texts). In diagnosing, the practitioner locates the abnormalities at work, and treats them directly, but also tries to identify and remove the abovementioned causes that led to the abnormalities. Getting rid of the cause helps reduce recurrences.

Western medicine attends to the cause to a small degree, as when it tries to reduce risk factors like smoking, risky sports (e.g. motorcycle-riding without a helmet), and a fat-laden diet. But MAV takes it much further. What would be considered healthy diets and lifestyle routines in modern medicine today – because no research has yet been done on their effects – are understood to cause the subtle abnormalities of *dosha*, *agni*, and *shrota* that over time lead to serious disease.

THE SIX STAGES OF PATHOGENESIS

The phrase 'over time' is crucial. MAV states that the three abnormalities give rise to disease in a sequential process. Disease develops through several stages, and it is only in the last stages that frank, objective signs of disease emerge. If, however, the clinician is alert enough to identify the disease in one of the early stages, a great deal of damage can be avoided. Almost as good as prevention is diagnosing a disease very early, so that the 'weed' can be nipped before its tendrils have crowded out more healthful flowers.

Before the fourth or fifth stage, symptoms may be nonexistent; and when they exist, they are so subtle that they seem 'merely' subjective. The heart's growing weakness may be masked until it becomes critical, as in a sudden heart attack. But patients may have been aware that *something* was wrong beforehand. Sometimes all they can say, though, is that they 'don't feel 100%'. Doctors, like patients, feel dissatisfied with returning a diagnosis of 'there's nothing wrong with

you', but they often feel they have little choice. Yet according to MAV, which avoids making a rigid distinction between mind and body, if the patient is moved to complain there must be something wrong. The stages of pathogenesis help one avoid dismissing such mysterious complaints, by letting one locate the hidden vitiation.

To understand the six stages of disease development, one must recall why the patient's feeling is considered so important for Ayurvedic diagnosis. It is because the mind and body are not separate entities, but a continuum. What straddles the apparent gap between them are the three *doshas*, and the subtle elements of the physiology such as *dhatus*, *shrotas*, and above all *ojas*. When these are balanced, immunity is at its strongest; when they are not, specific imbalances create specific illnesses. Ayurveda's analysis of disease formation is based on the *doshas*, *shrotas*, and another subtle entity that will be discussed, *ama*, the end-product of poor digestion.

Disease develops through a sequence of six stages involving not just the *doshas* but their five subdivisions, which have different functions in different parts of the body. For example, one of the subdivisions of *Pitta*, known as *ranjaka pitta*, is located in the red blood cells, liver, and spleen and governs blood formation.

A disease begins at stage one, *sancaya* or ('accumulation') with a *dosha* overaccumulating. The amount of one *dosha* increases beyond what it should be. The overaccumulation is brought on by some 'mistake' in diet, regimen, or thought. In our example of *ranjaka pitta*, the mistake might be that one eats too much *Pitta*-aggravating food during a hot summer.

In the second stage, 'aggravation' (*prakopa*), the accumulated *dosha* becomes aggravated, and develops the tendency to move to places other than where it belongs – in our example, places other than the blood, liver, and spleen.

In the third stage, 'dissemination' (*prasara*), the aggravated *dosha* begins to disseminate through the body: *ranjaka pitta* moves through the system.

In these first three stages no symptoms are felt at all. A skilled diagnostician can detect the imbalance all the same, by examining the pulse.

In the fourth stage, 'localization' (*sthana samshraya*), the wandering *dosha* settles somewhere other than where it belongs – usually in tissues to which it has a special affinity. In our example, aggravated *ranjaka pitta* has an affinity for the skin. This localization of the *dosha* occurs when the affected tissues have some obstruction in their circulatory channels (*shrotas*) due to *ama*, the product of poorly digested food.

At this stage, vague 'prodromal' symptoms emerge. The patient doesn't feel 100%, though he doesn't usually know what exactly is wrong or where the problem is. The skin may begin to feel itchy, but no clear disorder has arisen.

In the fifth stage, 'manifestation' (*vyakti*), objective signs arise: the skin might develop a rash. The likelihood of this stage emerging depends on the body type, climate, and season; the rash would be more likely to develop from the displacement of *ranjaka pitta* to the skin if the patient were a *Pitta* type, or if it were a tropical area, or if it were summertime.

In the sixth stage, 'disruption' (*bheda*), the disease erupts into its full fury. The rash may become extreme and disseminated. The disease now is harder to treat than at any earlier stage; at this stage it is firmly rooted in the physiology and may become chronic. That is why MAV places so much emphasis on early diagnosis.

How exactly do we diagnose early? MAV provides subtle diagnostic techniques that allow one to identify these stages.

MAV DIAGNOSTIC TECHNIQUES

Most of the effective Western diagnostic tools, such as biopsy or angiography, 'invade' the body. Even what we consider 'noninvasive' measures, such as X-rays and CAT-scans, invade the body with radiation, which does create a small level of risk (though its use may be necessary, of course). By contrast, MAV favors noninvasive diagnostic tools. While a doctor trained in MAV may use the entire array of Western diagnostic technologies, the MAV techniques add considerable subtlety and provide surprisingly thorough information. They serve not only to diagnose disease, but also to reveal the individual's state of balance, as well as the weak points of his or her physiology. Moreover, they are able to detect disease in the early stages we discussed above, so early that symptoms, even prodromal ones, have not yet arisen.

In addition to these techniques, MAV has classified hundreds of signs and symptoms (that are not clearly recognized in modern medicine) in terms of constitutional types. Many of these are features noted in modern medical practice by alert doctors but not as yet formally described. These include the body's, eyes', and joints' sizes and shapes, the distribution of fat under the skin, skin color and texture, hair color and texture, number and distribution of nevi (pigmented areas of the skin), the characteristics of nails, gait, rate of speech, tone of voice, gestures, speed of movement, strength of appetite, food preference, temperament, muscle tone and development, and many other features. A sense of some of these factors can be gained from our discussion of constitutional types in Chapter 5.

Classic Ayurvedic texts describe three main modalities of diagnosis: sight, speech, and touch. Sight includes careful examination for details of imbalance, which can be revealed in the eyes, tongue, and various other aspects of the physical structure. For example, look at your tongue in the mirror; if there is a lot of white 'fur' coating it, that may mean you are not digesting your food properly and are producing *ama*, the product of ill-digested food (see Chapter 7 for advice on correcting this).

Speech refers, of course, to the physician's interrogation, a process of questioning the patient about complaints, history, causative factors, etc. Aside from the insight into these afforded by MAV's theoretical framework, MAV further cautions doctors against discounting patients' complaints, for the reasons we have discussed.

Touch involves many aspects, such as palpation of the abdomen. In addition to feeling for abnormalities as in Western medicine, the Ayurvedic doctor is also checking for numerous characteristics of normal physiology which help to categorize the patient's state of health. The main approach through touch, however, is called pulse diagnosis; it is considered in MAV to be the best of all diagnostic tools.

Pulse diagnosis

In Chapter 2, we compared the body to a 'standing wave'; its solid appearance is only an illusion, and its reality is that it is a pattern of information and intelligence. A hologram – a two-dimensional object which, when laser light passes through, generates a three-dimensional image – is also more a pattern of knowledge than a collection of matter. A hologram has a fascinating property. Each individual point of the hologram contains all the information needed to construct the entire 3-D image. The body, too, if it is a pattern of intelligence rather than a heap of material, might be expected to contain enormous amounts of information about the whole in all or at least many of its parts. (This is of course true of DNA, for example.)

This analogy helps one understand why pulse diagnosis, or *nadi vigyan*, is so effective. Pulse diagnosis allows one to retrieve detailed information about the internal functioning of the body and its organs through signals present in the radial pulse. This information involves not only the cardiovascular system, but the other bodily systems as well. From the pulse, the diagnostician learns to gain information about the functioning of the bodily tissues, the state of the *doshas* and aggravation of the *doshas*, and much more, including, again, early stages of imbalance that precede full-blown symptoms.

According to MAV, pulse diagnosis works because the cardiovascular system, since it connects to every cell, can register what happens in them. The arteries, arterioles, and capillaries carry oxygen and nutrients to every cell in the body, and the system of veins returns the blood to the heart for replenishment – but all of them also convey information. While information is carried through the nervous system in the form of electrical impulses, it is carried in the cardiovascular system in the form of fluid vibratory waves. The waves which return through the veins all reach the heart, just as neural feedback collects in the brain. The waves then going out through the arteries give an overview of the total vibratory information which has collected in the heart. These subtle waves can be felt most easily above the arteries that are closest to the skin, such as the radial artery in the wrist (the same one that modern medicine uses to feel the pulse). Any imbalance creates a particular wave function, which can easily be identified by an experienced diagnostician.

At this point, no research has examined pulse diagnosis, but most clinicians who use it in their practice are quite impressed with the results. We have seen pulse diagnosis reveal things that are later confirmed by conventional tests: that the patient had trouble with kidney stones or hemorrhoids, atherosclerosis or liver trouble. Its accuracy, in the hands of an experienced

clinician can be remarkable. It is also helpful to the physician's bedside manner; attuning one's consciousness to the subtleties of the patient's pulse creates a moment of subtle, positive connection between doctor and patient. Again, though, the main value of pulse diagnosis is in revealing imbalances in the *doshas* and *subdoshas*, and the early stages of disease that result from such imbalances.

We do not think it appropriate to include instructions on how to do pulse diagnosis in this book. To master pulse diagnosis requires extensive training with an expert, who can point out subtle signs and give immediate feedback and correction. And a book certainly cannot teach the student how to do what a master diagnostician does: identify almost any disease, even when it is just starting to develop, from the pulse.

We can, however, mention a few rudiments. One takes the pulse from the radial artery of the right wrist of males and the left wrist of females. The physician's index, middle, and ring fingers are used for taking the pulse. Each finger relates to a specific *dosha*; the relative strength of pulsation under the finger tells you something about the *doshas* in that person. Also, each *dosha* has its characteristic style of pulsation. Ayurvedic tradition compares the pattern of the *Vata* pulse to the motion of a snake: light, quick, rough, thin, rapidly undulating. It compares *Pitta's* pulsating to a frog – sharp, cutting, jerky – and *Kapha's* to the motion of a swan: heavy, full, slow, soft, graceful. In time, the student becomes able to distinguish these three types of pulsation under the appropriate fingers; if they appear in the wrong finger, that tells one something about dislocation of the *doshas*. The pulse at the surface of the skin reflects imbalances present in the physiology, the *vikriti*; the pulse felt at a deeper level (one-half of the artery's thickness) is the *prakriti*, the underlying nature. Also, different parts of the fingertip relate to different *subdoshas*; and different techniques reveal information about the *dhatus*.

Standard training in pulse diagnosis involves, as a first exercise, monitoring one's own pulse. By doing so many times a day over a period, one becomes more alert to the subtle information carried by the pulse. In the course of a day, of a year, and of different types of activities, the three *doshas* vary in their predominance and their states of balance. As you monitor your own pulse, you become more alert to what, and how, your body is doing.

SUMMARY

MAV's understanding of pathogenesis focuses on the ground in which disease takes root. As such, it is a tremendous complement to the Western approach. It locates six stages through which disease develops, the earlier ones involving no overt symptoms at all; and it provides a wealth of subtle diagnostic techniques, which must be learned in the context of specialized professional training.

Doctors are no more satisfied with diagnoses of 'functional' or psychosomatic disease than patients are. And doctors take no pleasure in being unable to prevent recurrence, or prevent disease in the first place, or in seeing a heart attack fell an apparently healthy patient. The diagnostic techniques, and concept of pathogenesis, described above can help to improve our performance.

The above discussion has often referred to the importance of such factors as diet and routine in both causing and preventing illness. The next chapter discusses diet as a means of creating health.

7

Diet and digestion

According to the most ancient and venerated textbook of Ayurveda, the *Charaka Samhita*, 'The distinction between health and disease arises as the result of the difference between wholesome and unwholesome diet. . . . Disease is the result of faulty nutrition.' Along similar lines, perhaps, Hippocrates said: 'Leave your drugs in the pot at the pharmacy if you can't cure your patient with food.'

30 years ago, however, Hippocrates' professional descendants might have dismissed the idea. The notion that a change in diet could create health, in a way that had nothing to do with providing missing nutrients, was not considered scientific medicine. Medical opinion has shifted since then. It now recognizes diet as a risk factor in many diseases. For example, the American Cancer Society reports that at least 35% of America's 900 000 new cases of cancer per year have diet as a significant risk factor. It is also known that a diet rich in the wrong kinds of fat creates a higher risk of coronary disease, the number one killer in the US today. As a result of such findings, contemporary medicine has become more interested in the potential medical role of diet.

But modern knowledge of how eating influences health remains preliminary. As clinicians practicing Maharishi Ayur-Veda (MAV), we have seen several cases that Hippocrates might have applauded: before we had a chance to apply a treatment program, a patient's condition resolved simply from a suggested dietary change. We know of almost no parallel in contemporary medicine, for example, to a patient who, after ten specialists had failed to find any cause or cure for her severe headaches, was cured simply by adopting the diet recommended by her MAV doctor. We have seen scores of similar instances. MAV's dietary concerns go well beyond using diet to address disease conditions and avoiding dietary factors that cause disease: it also aims to use diet to optimize health and well-being in the positive sense.

All of this suggests that MAV's knowledge of diet has much to contribute to Western medicine. This knowledge is organized around four major principles. The first we have already implied: that diet can be a therapeutic modality. It is not merely an adjunct to other treatments, but plays a critical and sometimes primary role in treatment, and is central to MAV's approach to prevention. Western medical research is beginning to find some evidence for food as therapy, having found dietary factors to help in such areas as preventing peptic ulcer relapse (Hills 1990), and reducing rheumatoid arthritis (Darlington et al 1986, Hicklin et al 1989, Skoldstam et al 1979, Uden et al 1983, Stroud 1983, Hafstrom et al 1988), cardiovascular risk, and hypertension (Beilin 1987), but MAV takes the idea much, much further. The influence of food is so subtle that the Vedic science of pharmacology, *dravyaguna*, analyzes food in the same sophisticated way that it analyzes medicines. It makes no distinction between food and medicine – they are considered one category, not two.

The second principle is that a food's taste is not a mere decoration, but has nutritional meaning. This chapter will explain how patients can use their sense of taste to ensure nutritional balance.

The third principle is that different people respond differently to the same foods, and, conversely, that different foods suit different people. The food essayist M. F. K. Fischer wrote that 'such a thing as an egg can be manna to one person and a searing time bomb to another'. MAV provides a framework for understanding and using this fact of nature, to which Western nutrition has not yet paid much attention. *Everyone*, it tends to say, should take only *x* grams of fat or at least *y* grams of protein (with a few medical exceptions). MAV, by contrast, systematically analyzes why the food that benefits one person can harm another.

The fourth principle is that as important as what one eats is how one *digests* it. A patient complaining that his digestion is sluggish or weak would not be a candidate for Western treatment; medical training prepares us only to treat fully formed diseases, such as ulcers or colitis. Yet MAV holds that sluggish or weak digestion is a significant pathogenic factor, and that an optimal diet would be not only useless, but even harmful, if it were not properly digested.

Below we look in more detail at each of these four principles.

PRINCIPLE 1: FOOD CAN BE THERAPY

In the West, we are used to thinking of the body as matter operating according to Newtonian physical laws. This is more or less how we think of food – as matter in the form of protein, vitamins, carbohydrates, lipids, and minerals. For that reason, unless the patient lacks a specific vitamin, mineral, or other micronutrient, we would not expect food to have a specific value in treating disease. We would not expect, for example, that a change to a *Vata*-pacifying diet could rid a patient of chronic headaches, or that a *Kapha*-pacifying diet could cure allergies.

Yet MAV has successfully treated such diseases in just such ways – with changes of diet unrelated to nutritional deficits. MAV holds that the body is more than matter – it is a dynamic pattern, a network of information and intelligence – and this is how it understands the influence of herbs: as 'tuning forks' that enliven the underlying pattern and sequence of natural law that prevails in a healthy body. Correct diet is understood in the same way. Food, too, is a network of energy and intelligence. Properly chosen food can contribute to keeping the body's dynamic patterns in a state of balance. It adds not only material and energy, but also *order* to a system that is constantly resisting the disordering influence of entropy (Schrödinger 1967). Maintaining the body's balance and order is considered the basis of health; using diet as a means for this is a crucial way of improving a person's health (or, if ignored, of worsening it).

In this chapter, we will explain several key factors used to find the diet that best promotes health for a given individual. Among them are approaches traditionally emphasized by MAV, such as *prakriti*, digestive strength, and taste groups.

PRINCIPLE 2: A FOOD'S TASTE IS A GUIDE TO ITS NUTRITIONAL VALUE

The essence of MAV's use of diet is in applying a principle discussed in Chapter 5: balancing the individual's three *doshas*. But the exact state of doshic balance, the *deha prakriti*, changes from time to time, and the state of current imbalance, the *vikriti*, changes from day to day: today there is more *Vata*, tomorrow *Pitta* is a little aggravated. The climate, the state of one's work and one's home life – everything one does and experiences – can alter the current state of balance. As that state of balance changes, so does the ideal diet.

Consider a woman who is by *deha prakriti* a *Pitta/Vata*. Her underlying *prakriti* has more *Pitta* than *Vata*, and less of *Kapha* than either of the other two. But on a hot summer day, her *Pitta* will overaccumulate; if she has also been straining at work, her *Vata* becomes aggravated too. *Kapha* remains low, however. Her ideal diet today would pacify *Pitta* primarily, *Vata* to a lesser extent, and *Kapha* not at all. But in the winter, when *Vata* tends to be aggravated, the main purpose of her diet will probably be to pacify *Vata*; *Pitta* will need less attention.

How can we determine what is preferable today for a given patient? According to MAV, patients ultimately can regain the ability to make their own determinations, and spontaneously at that. This is accomplished above all by becoming more alert to the information conveyed by the sense of taste.

This may seem, to a Western clinician, uncomfortably subjective; and there is no denying that the modern understanding of vitamins and minerals has made a major contribution to the field of nutrition. But nutritionists have repeatedly stated that our understanding of nutrients is sketchy. How does science determine what 'recommended daily allowances' are? The main methods are by depriving laboratory animals of a given nutrient until they develop diseases, or by observing people who already have deficiencies. This emphasis on abnormal states has skewed our view of nutrition. We think of it in too simple terms: at least a certain number of milligrams of calcium per day, no more than a certain number of milligrams of vitamin D. This can be valuable, but needs to go further, since it ignores not only the antioxidant role of certain nutrients, but also the fact that the human body is an intricate ecosystem. Food affects the balance of every area of the body. MAV holds, in fact, that the ideal diet would suit an individual as precisely as a key fits a lock.

Why would a subtle and natural sense of what the body needs be rooted in the sense of taste? In a natural environment, taste (and smell) lead animals towards the nutrients they need – if not infallibly, still to an impressive degree. Similarly, human beings for ages relied on taste to avoid toxic or unhealthy foods and to find nutritious ones; the sweet tooth, a human universal, was historically useful because it led people to nutrient-bearing fruit. Some research on adults suggests that unconscious cues for nutrient choice keep nutrient intake constant (Wurtman et al 1985). Pregnant women's food aversions or 'morning sickness' are coming to be understood as a mechanism to protect the embryo from the abortifacients (toxins that induce abortion) and teratogens (toxins that cause birth defects) that may be present in foods – and these food aversions and cravings are all based on the foods' taste and smell (Profet 1992). Such research supports the view that taste is not just a decoration, but is deeply connected to the nutritive value of food. Thus the rationale for the MAV approach: taste is our most natural connection to food. Yet modern nutritionists have, surprisingly, ignored it so far. Ayurveda's approach to restoring our natural alertness to taste may supplement the as yet incomplete knowledge of dietetics.

Taste groups

MAV classifies all foods as belonging to one (or more) of six taste groups. The six tastes are sweet (*madhura*), sour (*amla*), salty (*lavana*), pungent (*katu*), bitter (*tikta*) and astringent (*kashaya*). Some of these are easy to define: there is never any question about what constitutes a salty taste. Others need a little more explanation. For example, 'sweet' includes not only sugary foods but also milk, grains (like wheat, rice, and barley), bread, cooked starchy tubers (potatoes and sweet potatoes), some cooked vegetables, and sweet fruits. 'Sour' includes not only lemons and other sour citrus fruits but also yogurt, cheese, other curdled milk products, fermented substances, carbonated beverages, and tomatoes. 'Pungent' means hot and spicy. Examples of 'bitter' are turmeric, eggplant, zucchini, and green

Box 7.1 The six taste groups: some examples

Sweet

- Most grains like wheat, rice, barley, corn, etc.; most bread.
- Most legumes, such as beans, lentils and peas (contain some sweet taste).
- Milk and sweet milk products, such as cream, butter, and ghee.
- Sweet fruits like dates, figs, grapes, pears, mangos.
- Certain cooked vegetables, especially starchy tubers: potato, sweet potato, carrot, beet.
- Sugar in any form (but not honey, which also has an astringent taste).

Sour

- Sour fruits like lemon, lime, sour oranges, etc.
- Sour milk products like yogurt, cheese, sour cream, and whey.
- Fermented substances (other than cultured milk products) like wine, vinegar, soy sauce, sour cabbage, etc.

Salty

- Any kind of salt (e.g. sea salt, rock salt).
- Foods to which large amounts of salt are added (pickles, chips, etc.).

Pungent

- Spices like chili, black pepper, mustard seeds, ginger, cumin, garlic, etc.
- Certain vegetables like radish, onion, etc.

Bitter

- Certain fruits, like olives, grapefruits, etc.
- Green, leafy vegetables like spinach, green cabbage, brussel sprouts, zucchini.
- Eggplant, bitter gourd, chicory.
- Certain spices, like fenugreek and turmeric.

Astringent

- Legumes, beans, lentils.
- Walnuts, hazelnuts.
- Honey.
- Sprouts, lettuce and other green, leafy vegetables, rhubarb, most raw vegetables.
- Pomegranate, apples (to some degree), berries, persimmons, cashew, and unripe fruits (contain some astringence).

leafy vegetables like spinach. 'Astringent' includes foods that have a drying quality, such as beans, pomegranates and apples. A list of foods in different taste groups is given in Box 7.1.

As to how one applies this classification, the most basic rule is simple: include something from each taste group in every meal. This is necessary both for providing complete nutrition and for keeping the *doshas* balanced.

Why is such a simple rule – when combined with several other Ayurvedic principles – considered so important in ensuring balanced nutrition? For one thing, the six tastes stimulate, among them, the proper sequence of the digestive process. Also, human beings, by biodesign, seek dietary diversity; this both ensures adequate nutrition and reduces overexposure to one food. None the less, this natural tendency can be dulled in modern society; between habit, Madison Avenue, and stress, the body's natural preferences are overridden. For example, the typical American diet underrepresents the pungent, bitter, and astringent tastes, and overemphasizes the sweet taste, as well as the salty and sour. These three tastes increase *Kapha dosha*, which is part of how MAV would explain the prevalence of obesity (a *Kapha* imbalance) in the West.

This points to a deeper reason for a concern with food's taste: according to MAV, the taste groups indicate food's more fundamental qualities. Each taste has a potent effect on each *dosha*, to either increase or decrease it. Sweet, sour, and salty tastes decrease *Vata* and increase *Kapha*. Pungent, bitter, and astringent tastes increase *Vata* and reduce *Kapha*. The sweet, bitter, and astringent tastes decrease *Pitta*; and the sour, salty and pungent tastes increase *Pitta*. In this is the rationale behind many of the dietary recommendations in the *dosha*-specific diets given below. For example, since the sweet taste reduces *Vata*, and the astringent increases it, *Vata* types should take relatively more sweet and fewer astringent foods, although they need *some* of both (Table 7.1).

The tastes are said each to represent predominant *mahabhutas*. We discussed the five *mahabhutas* in Chapter 5 as being the precursors of the *doshas*, and as possibly being equivalent to quantum spin types. Of the six tastes, sweet is dominated by earth and water (*prithivi* and *jala*), sour by earth and fire (*prithivi* and *tejas*), salty by water and fire (*jala* and *tejas*), pungent by air and fire (*vayu* and *tejas*), bitter by air and space (*vayu* and *akasha*), and astringent by air and earth (*vayu* and *prithivi*) (Table 7.2).

Table 7.1 How the tastes affect the *doshas*

Sweet, sour, salty	Increase *Kapha*, decrease *Vata*
Pungent, bitter, astringent	Decrease *Kapha*, increase *Vata*
Pungent, sour, salty	Increase *Pitta*
Sweet, bitter, astringent	Decrease *Pitta*

Table 7.2 The six tastes (*rasas*) and their relation to the five *mahabhutas*

Rasa	Predominant *mahabhutas*
Sweet	*Prithivi* and *jala*
Sour	*Prithivi* and *tejas*
Salty	*Jala* and *tejas*
Pungent	*Vayu* and *tejas*
Bitter	*Vayu* and *akasha*
Astringent	*Vayu* and *Prithivi*

This explains how it is that the tastes affect the *doshas*, for the *doshas* are made of combinations of *mahabhutas*. *Vata*, for example, is made of the combination of *akasha* and *vayu*. Thus bitter foods (*vayu* and *akasha*) aggravate it, as do pungent and astringent foods, all of which contain *vayu*. Similarly, *Pitta* is made of *tejas* and *jala*; thus the salty taste (*tejas* and *jala*) aggravates it, as do the sour taste (which contains *tejas*) and pungent taste (which contains *tejas*). As for *Kapha*, it is made of *prithivi* and *jala*; thus the sweet taste (which contains the same two *mahabhutas*) aggravates it, as do sour and salty tastes, which contain *prithivi* and *jala* respectively.

This is an example of the Ayurvedic law that was covered in the *dosha* chapters: the law of similars and opposites. A quality is increased by similars, and reduced by opposites. Thus a *dosha* made up of two specific *mahabhutas* is increased by foods that emphasize those two *mahabhutas*, and decreased by foods in which other *mahabhutas* prevail.

Some other nutritionally significant qualities of food

It is important to note that MAV considers other aspects of food that affect the doshic balance. Among these are food's *virya* or potency – whether it is heating (*ushna*) or cooling (*sheeta*);* its qualities or *gunas* – whether it is rough or smooth, cold, hot, light, heavy, dry, oily, stable or mobile, soft or hard, etc.; its *vipaka* – its aftertaste or delayed effect (sweet, sour, or pungent); and its unique qualities (known as *prabhava*).

The term *guna* here refers to something different

from the three *gunas* discussed in Chapter 4. Those three, *sattwa*, *rajas*, and *tamas*, are non-material, operating in the realm of consciousness and the mind. But these *gunas*, of which there are 20, are considered to be qualities of matter. They are used in discussing such material phenomena as weather, behavior, herbs, and *prakriti/vikriti* as well as food. For an example of a behavior and its effect on the *gunas*, staying awake through the night is said to increase roughness (*khara*).

The *gunas* exist in pairs, three of which in particular are commonly used in evaluating food: heavy and light (*guru* and *laghu*); cold and hot (*sheeta* and *ushna*); and oily and dry (*snigdha* and *rooksha*). These qualities are also natural signals of nutritional value. One central way of applying these is by noting that heavy food is harder to digest than light food. When digestive capacity is low, the person must be careful to favor lighter food; even people with normal digestion can overload the digestive system with too much heavy food. As shown below, the results will be unhealthy products of the digestive process. Common 'heavy' foods include meat, and oily and fatty food; indeed, these have all been implicated in heart disease, cancer and other chronic disorders. (We will return to this in the section on dairy products and vegetarianism.)

Food of certain *gunas* is said to affect the *doshas* as well (Table 7.3).

Thus, MAV does not suggest that we rely only on taste, but it does hold that taste is the most important of the many factors involved in balancing the diet. It is also the simplest to apply.

No matter what one's type, all six tastes should be represented at every meal. On the other hand, the balance of tastes ideal for an individual depends on his or

Table 7.3 Some examples of the pairs of *gunas*, and how they affect the *doshas*

Heavy (*guru*) K↑, V↓	Light (*laghu*) V↑, K↓
Cold (*sheeta*) K↑, VP↓	Hot (*ushna*) P↑, VK↓
Oily (*snigdha*) K↑, V↓	Dry (*rooksha*) V↑, K↓

Note: The above three pairs of *gunas* are the ones most commonly used in discussing food's effects on the *doshas*. The other pairs of *gunas* include: soft (*mridu*) and hard (*kathina*); clear (*vishada*) and viscous (*pichhila*); rough (*khara*) and smooth (*mrisana*); gross (*sthula*) and subtle (*sookshma*); semi-solid (*sandra*) and liquid (*drava*); stable (*sthira*) and unstable (*sara*).

---

*Some Ayurvedic sources refer to eight types of *virya*: hot, cold, light, heavy, unctuous, nonunctuous, dull, and sharp. MAV, however, uses the two-type classification.

her body type. *Vatas* need relatively more sweet, sour, and salty food, because these tastes pacify *Vata*; *Pittas* need more sweet and less sour food.

PRINCIPLE 3: THE PREDOMINANT FUNCTIONAL *DOSHA* SHOULD DETERMINE WHICH FOOD IS BEST FOR A GIVEN PATIENT

MAV considers several factors, such as the season (Ch. 9), the strength of the 'digestive fire' or *agni*, and specific physiological conditions, in determining the ideal diet for a given individual. But the most important is the individual's mix of *doshas*, since the best clue to what foods one needs is the current state of imbalance, or *vikriti*. *Deha prakriti* matters as well: as we have seen, a person with a particular constitutional type is most likely to overaccumulate the *dosha* which dominates his or her *prakriti*. A *Vata* person, for example, is most likely to develop *Vata* imbalances. But *Pittas* and *Kaphas* can develop *Vata* ailments also. The possible variations are numerous, and thus *vikriti* is the best guide.

As this suggests, the three diets given in Appendix 1 of this chapter are not meant to be applied rigidly – one should mix them if this is appropriate. But many people find that following them carefully for a while helps develop a feeling for how food influences the body. For example, the list below shows that barley reduces *Kapha*. In our current environment, even *Kapha* predominants would not normally have a yen for barley. Instead, they might crave a hot fudge sundae – an unfortunate choice for their *Kapha*-dominated physiology. After following these diets for a while, though, several *Kaphas* have told us that they no longer like ice cream and fudge (or at least that they associate sundaes with feeling heavy and congested, and thus lose their taste for them); some even find themselves hankering after barley. Following the diet helped reconnect their palates with their nutritional needs.

This is not to say that *prakriti* and *vikriti* is completely ignored in spontaneous diet choices by those not trained in MAV. Why does one person put so much sugar in her tea, when another drinks his black? Such questions are often obvious once you understand constitutional types and how food affects the *doshas*.

The law of similars and opposites revisited

This simple law – similars increase similars, opposites decrease opposites – is employed in Ayurveda's dietary advice for pacifying *Vata*, *Pitta* and *Kapha* doshas. A purely *Vata* person needs warmer, sweeter, oilier foods, because they settle his or her *Vata dosha*. (*Vata dosha* is dry, cold, and astringent, so foods with the opposite qualities such as sweet, warm, and oily settle it.) For a *Kapha*, such foods will lead to weight gain and lethargy, since these foods increase *Kapha*. A purely *Kapha* person thrives on spicy, pungent foods, which reduce *Kapha*. These foods help him or her keep weight down and sinuses clear. The same foods, however, will be disastrous for a *Pitta* person. A *Pitta* is hot enough already without adding peppers and spices, which inflame *Pitta* even more. If a *Pitta* does favor those kinds of food, it may lead to too much intestinal heat and excess stomach acid, as well as to outbursts of anger. Appendix 1 to this chapter lists diets that pacify each of the three *doshas*.

Note that we must also consider the season before we come to a conclusion on what diet is best for an individual. For example, a *Vata* predominant may have to take into consideration a more *Pitta*-reducing diet during the heat of the summer. Chapter 9 summarizes when to use what diet, depending on predominant *dosha* and season.

What does one do if, like most people, one is a mixed *vikriti*? A simple answer is to mix the dietary advice given above. A *Vata/Pitta*, for example, should pay attention to both *doshas*' diets, giving more emphasis to the *Vata* diet in the windy, *Vata*-increasing cold of winter and to the *Pitta* diet in the *Pitta*-aggravating heat of summer (for autumn and spring, and for other types, Chapter 9 gives details).

Again, these diets are not meant to be rigid. The body itself is the best Ayurvedic authority. The advice in this chapter will help to re-establish contact, to develop truly natural eating habits by being alert to what the body is telling us.

PRINCIPLE 4: HOW ONE EATS IS AS IMPORTANT AS WHAT ONE EATS

Recall the way most people feel after Thanksgiving

dinner. This is an extreme case, but clinical experience suggests that the standard American diet, with its heavy protein, sugar, and fat content, can be hard on the digestive tract. To MAV, these digestive burdens are not merely nuisances. Poorly digested food, MAV tells us, produces more than just discomfort. If food is not digested well, even if the food itself is full of nutrients, the end-product of digestion can have insidious effects.

In MAV terms, the end-product of those meals that leave one feeling comfortable, light, and fresh is the substance we referred to in Chapter 4, *ojas*, which sustains all the *dhatus*, the principles upholding the bodily tissues. *Ojas* not only nourishes all the body tissues, it also strengthens immunity, and produces a feeling of happiness.

Ama

The end-product of poorly digested food is called *ama*. *Ama* is said to clog the channels in the body (the *shrotas*), giving rise to disease. *Ama*, clogging the *shrotas*, can cause lethargy, dullness, and heaviness. Worse, it is a precursor of illness – MAV considers it a central culprit in pathogenesis. Although *ama*'s equivalent in modern medicine is not yet clear, it is well known in Western medicine that circulating toxins usually originate in the digestive system. Because *ama* contributes to the early stage of many diseases, MAV considers reducing *ama* to be a crucial concern of any physician.

The *agni*

A central element in preventing *ama* is what MAV calls the 'fire' or *agni*. MAV, as we saw in Chapter 5, identifies 13 *agnis* governing different aspects of the digestive process and parts of the body (for example, a series of different *agnis* convert one *dhatu* into the next one). But the most important *agni* is what we have called the *digestive fire*, called in Sanskrit the *jatharagni*. The digestive fire is second only to *vikriti* as a factor determining the body's dietary needs. 'Digestive fire' refers to the digestive system's overall ability to digest food; it is equivalent to digestive enzymes. Some people have a powerful *agni*, others a weak one, and most people fall somewhere in between or have *agnis* that

vary. Those with a particularly powerful *agni* – a 'cast-iron stomach' – need not be as careful about the dietary suggestions that follow, although they will benefit from them. But if the *agni* is average, and particularly if it is weak (for those who must 'eat like a bird' to avoid a bloated feeling), the suggestions given below will be crucial. The more they attend to them, the better their digestion will be. They are especially helpful for patients with functional digestive problems – a bloated feeling after eating, a tendency toward eructation or flatulence, or aggravated hiatal hernias – but their significance is far greater in that they prevent *ama*, which is considered central to pathogenesis.

The strength of the *agni* is to some extent related to *vikriti* and *prakriti*: *Vatas* tend to have variable *agnis*, *Pittas* strong or sharp *agnis* – which in themselves are not necessarily healthy – and *Kaphas* slow or dull *agnis*. This general principle must be applied flexibly to most patients, who usually have mixed predominant *doshas*.

Dietary advice

The tips for ideal digestion may appear at first glance to be rules one must discipline oneself to follow. But they are not meant in that spirit. Rather, they are techniques for 'deprogramming'. They are meant to help free one from inappropriate habits and foster one's attentiveness to what the body is signaling. When we looked at the diets for different *doshas*, we considered the question of *what* to eat. The following suggestions will tell us three more things: (1) when to eat; (2) how much to eat; (3) how to eat.

When to eat

1. Eat the main meal around noon time, when the digestive fire is strongest. This is discussed in more detail in Chapter 9, in the section on daily routine. Breakfast and dinner should be lighter.

2. Don't eat again until the previous meal is fully digested. This usually takes at least two and a half hours (for *Pitta* types), and can take longer. As one Ayurvedic *vaidya* (physician) put it, eating before the previous meal is digested is like adding raw beans into a soup in which a previous batch has been cooking. The soup never gets quite done. It is the same with

digestion – we strain the digestive system if we eat small snacks all day long. Eating while the stomach is still digesting results in *ama*, the end-product of poor digestion. This topic is also discussed in more detail in Chapter 9.

3. Attend to your level of hunger. The signal that the previous meal has been digested is the appearance of hunger. Before eating, one should pay attention to that signal. Are you really hungry, or are you just eating to satisfy an emotional need, a craving, or a habit? On the other hand, if you feel hungry, your body is asking to be fed.

4. Keep regular meal times. A regular routine helps the body digest better. The body is a sophisticated timepiece, and it runs better if we attune ourselves to its natural cycles. For most people, lunch should usually be somewhere between 11 a.m. and 1 p.m., and dinner between 5 and 6.30 p.m.

How much to eat

Eat to three-quarters of your capacity. The reason a bloated feeling is unpleasant is that it is a complaint from the body. MAV tries to prevent it by having us eat not to 100% of capacity, and certainly not above it, but to 75%.

Ayurveda considers 75% to be roughly equivalent to the amount of food two hands, cupped, could hold. It is considered healthy because it allows the *agni* (modern medicine would say 'digestive enzymes') room to work. This allows digestion to be complete.

The signal that one has reached three-quarters of capacity is that one feels satisfied but not full. Feeling full means that one has gone to 100% of capacity and the food is distending the stomach (feeling 'stuffed' is another step beyond this). At three-quarters of capacity, one feels satisfied, but light and easy in the abdomen, without any feeling of pressure.

How to eat

1. Eat in a settled atmosphere. Stopping at a drive-in, grabbing a sandwich, and devouring it while hurrying through traffic may be a common activity today, but MAV would argue that it is neither natural nor healthy. Subjectively, people may notice that in those circumstances the food does not feel as comfortable going down as it does when they sit down and eat in a settled atmosphere.

It is preferable, according to MAV, not to divide one's attention during the meal. In other words, it is better not to read, work, drive, or watch TV during meals, and just to enjoy the taste of the food.

2. Don't eat when upset. If one is upset, disturbed or angry at meal time, it is best to postpone the meal for a little while.

Earlier we discussed how emotions influence our physiology. This is especially true when we eat. Food rebuilds the body; and our feelings when we take in that food affect our biochemistry directly, and through it the quality of our digestion and the products of digestion, which in turn affect the whole structure of the body.

Meal time should be a time free from arguments, a time to just enjoy, either alone or in the warmth of family and friends. This, by the way, is one value of the traditional practice of saying grace or a blessing at the beginning of a meal: to create a tranquil, harmonious feeling at the table before eating.

3. Always sit down to eat.

4. Don't talk while chewing food. Chewing well and swallowing before speaking help predigest the food.

5. Avoid taking milk with meals that have mixed tastes. Ayurveda traditionally considers cow's milk to be a particularly healthy food, but it also gives a number of rules for optimizing digestion of milk. We discuss milk in some detail near the end of this chapter, and give some MAV advice on its proper use. The above rule is an example of what is covered there. One should especially avoid combining milk with fish, meat, banana, and spicy, salty, or sour foods, for these combinations make the milk more difficult to digest. (One favorite American breakfast combination, milk and orange juice, is not healthy by Ayurvedic standards. The sourness of the orange juice tends to curdle the milk and make it harder to digest. Many people have sensed this incompatibility at times.) Milk combines well, however, with toast, sweet fruits, cereals, or any other food from the sweet taste group. It is also acceptable to take milk at least 30 minutes away from a larger meal.

6. Favor fresh, wholesome foods. According to

Ayurveda, leftover food loses some of its enlivening and organizing power, and becomes harder to digest. It is, for these reasons, less valuable for health. Ayurveda recommends favoring freshly prepared foods.

By wholesome foods Ayurveda means using the best possible quality of ingredients in preparing food. Organically grown foods, which are untainted by free-radical-producing pesticides and chemical fertilizers, are especially recommended when possible.

7. In general, favor cooked foods over raw ones. Cooked foods are easier to digest, because cooking is a first step in the process of digestion. The oven's heat does some of the work that the digestive fire would otherwise have to do. The heat breaks down complex protein, fat, and carbohydrate structures that our own body would, if we ate the food raw, need to break down itself; it can also denature toxins.

This rule, like all the others, is not meant to be applied rigidly. Most people prefer to eat fruit raw, for example – although Ayurveda holds that ripe fruit has already been cooked by the sun.

Some raw food advocates maintain that cooking results in minor losses of nutrients. Such losses in cooking will be more than compensated for, because the body will find the remaining nutrients easier to assimilate. Of course, food should not be overcooked. Taste is usually a good guide.

8. Avoid cold drinks. With meals, sip moderate amounts of warm or room temperature water. Cold drinks douse the digestive fire; in Western terms, they reduce the optimal functioning of the cells in the stomach which produce the digestive enzymes. Moderate amounts of water (not cold in either case) with a meal help liquify the food for easier digestion. (Too much liquid before or during the meal, however, dilutes the digestive enzymes.) In very hot weather, cool drinks are all right, especially for those with *Pitta* constitutions. But they should not be *cold*, that is, served with ice or taken straight from the refrigerator. Don't drink a lot of water or any liquid just before, during, or just after a meal, as this can drown the digestive fire and slow the digestion.

9. After eating, take 4 or 5 minutes to sit quietly. Don't eat and run, at least not without a 4- or 5-minute buffer period. This will allow digestion to begin effortlessly.

PURIFYING VERSUS BALANCING DIETS

Another way of classifying individualized diets is according to the patient's need for a balancing or a purifying diet. Balancing diets are the three covered above – the *Vata*, *Pitta*, and *Kapha* diets – which are, of course, customized to suit the patient's unique mix of *doshas*. The purifying diet is appropriate when the physician determines that a large amount of *ama* and other toxins have accumulated. It involves lighter, easier to digest foods in smaller quantities; these let the digestive fire not only avoid the production of new *ama*, but also remove pre-existing *ama*. The physician determines the presence of *ama* through examination of the pulse, of the tongue (which is covered with a sticky white 'fuzz' when *ama* is accumulating), and of other factors.

The *ama*-reducing diet is designed to gently clear away impurities by increasing the power of *jatharagni*, the digestive fire. When the *agni* is strong, it is said to burn away existing pockets of *ama* and prevent new impurities from building up.

Note that the effectiveness of fasting as a treatment for rheumatoid arthritis, demonstrated in modern medical research (Stroud 1983, Skoldstam et al 1979), corresponds to the MAV understanding of that disease as being caused by *ama*; fasting is used only with great care in MAV because it can weaken the *dhatus* and tissues, but it does reduce accumulated *ama*. For most situations, however, the use of the purifying diet is far preferable as a way to reduce *ama*.

To follow the purifying diet:

- Favor
  - light grain: Couscous, rye, millet, or quinoa
  - cooked, fresh vegetables
  - salty lassi (see appendix to this chapter for instructions on how to make it)
  - fruit
- Avoid heavy foods such as yeasted breads, pasta, potatoes, and desserts.

The *ama*-reducing diet is nourishing yet light and easy to digest. To understand how this diet can reduce *ama*, think of digestion as a kind of furnace. Throwing too much fuel on the fire snuffs it out. This is what happens when one eats foods that are too heavy, eats food at the wrong time, or eats before one has completely digested the previous meal. Digestion gets overwhelmed, and instead of getting processed correctly, the food putrefies and creates impurities that collect in the body, weigh it down, and cause disease.

When it is burning strongly, the digestive fire not only digests food completely, preventing *ama* from being formed, but it is said to burn off the *ama* that is already accumulated. The lighter diet recommended allows the digestive *agni* to revive itself. Once the *agni* is stronger, the patient can gradually add heavier foods to his or her diet, just as one might start a fire with small kindling and gradually feed in the larger logs.

It is important to note that, when not weighed down by too much food or the wrong kinds of food, the body removes *ama* with its own self-cleaning mechanisms. It naturally eliminates impurities through the bowels, bladder, and skin. It even has mechanisms to dissolve clots in the legs or plaque in the arteries. Research has shown that blockages in the arteries can be removed through a program of meditation, diet, exercise, and healthier lifestyle (Ornish et al 1990).

SOME SPECIFIC DIETARY ADVICE
Why MAV values certain dairy products

Ghee

Ghee is . . . good for the eyes, stimulant for digestion, supports glow and beauty, enhances memory and stamina, promotes longevity, and protects the body from various diseases.'

Bhavaprakash, a major Ayurvedic text

Ghee is butter from which the water (about 20% of butter) and milk solids have been removed. It has a very long shelf life (it can last for years) and a pleasing flavor. Ayurveda has traditionally considered ghee to be one of the most health-promoting of all foods. Ghee is said to pacify all three of the *doshas*, strengthen the body, improve memory and mental functions, and promote longevity. Ghee stimulates the digestive fire if taken with a meal. One teaspoon per meal is considered about right; too much ghee will douse the digestive fire (2 tablespoons of ghee per day is considered the maximum; too much ghee increases *Kapha* and can clog the system).

In addition to dietary use, ghee has numerous medical applications. It is useful, for example, applied topically on burns. Taken internally, it is considered helpful to the eyes. It is used in some important MAV herbal mixtures; in these preparations it serves as a vehicle that carries important chemicals and antioxidants past lipid-permeable cell membranes and into the cells.

The great benefits MAV sees in ghee can seem odd to Westerners. After all, ghee contains a great deal of fatty acids. However, closer examination shows that recent understandings in nutrition strongly support the MAV view. To understand why, we must examine the nature of fatty foods.

Fats fall into two categories: saturated and unsaturated. The saturated fats are of two kinds: long-chain and short-chain fatty acids. Short-chain fatty acids are assimilated, absorbed, and then metabolized so that they release energy. Long-chain fatty acids, by contrast, are not completely metabolized and are associated with cancer and blood-clots (thrombosis). Most animal fat consists of long-chain fatty acids. As for unsaturated fatty acids, they can be either monounsaturated or polyunsaturated. The monounsaturated fats are very healthy; the polyunsaturates were once considered so, but are now known to be the opposite. The reason involves the kind of chemical bonds these fats form. Monounsaturated fats form single bonds, but the polyunsaturated fats form multiple bonds; and the multiple bonds are places where oxidation of the fatty acids occur, which makes the fats toxic. For example, foods fried in polyunsaturated fatty acids such as vegetable oils become oxidized, making them unhealthy for consumption (Hageman et al 1991). (Oxidation is a process where there is a loss of electrons, which affects double bonds in fatty acids, so that they become injurious to the body; during this process of oxidation, there is generation of free radicals, which are also harmful to the body, as discussed in the next chapter.) Thus polyunsaturated fatty acids have been associated with the onset of cancer and with physiological damage caused by oxidized lipids. Most vegetable oils contain predominantly polyunsaturated fatty acids and are therefore not advisable for consumption (an exception is sesame oil, which contains powerful antioxidants). Commercially sold margarine and other hydrogenated fats are especially unhealthy; they contain 30–40%

trans fatty acids, many of which do not occur in nature (Willet & Ascherio 1994), and have been shown to increase low-density lipoprotein (LDL, the 'bad' cholesterol) as much as saturated fats do (Mensink & Katan 1990). Also, several epidemiological studies have found a positive association of trans fatty acids and coronary heart disease (Willet & Ascherio 1994).

By contrast to polyunsaturated fatty acids, the monounsaturated fatty acids are associated with prevention of heart disease and cancer. Some oils contain predominantly monounsaturated fatty acids, notably olive oil, mustard oil, canola oil, and rapeseed oil.

With this background we can understand why ghee might be considered very healthy even from a Western perspective (Sharma 1990). For one thing, most of its saturated fats are short-chain fatty acids, and only a small percentage are long-chain fatty acids (11%). For another, ghee contains up to 27% monounsaturated fatty acids, and only 4–5% polyunsaturated fatty acids. Finally, the human body requires intake of both saturated and unsaturated fatty acids, and ghee comes closest to having the right ratio of these types of acids (about 60–66% saturated fats, mostly short-chain fatty acids, and 27% monounsaturated fats). In addition, ghee has other benefits. It contains 2–3% conjugated linoleic acid (Aneja & Murthi 1991), a chemical that may have anticarcinogenic properties, as well as a considerable number of antioxidants (free radical scavengers) and vitamins A, D, E, and K. And ghee itself is not very susceptible to oxidation (Nath & Rama Murthy 1988), which is partly why its shelf life is so long.

Does ghee raise cholesterol levels in the body? A loosely constructed epidemiological study argued so (Jacobson 1987), but it drew scientific criticism (Nath & Rama Murthy 1988). More recently, a tighter experimental study showed the opposite. A 10% ghee diet given to experimental rats for a period of four weeks did not have any significant effect on blood cholesterol (Crosser et al 1994).

Ghee is made by two main methods: either from butter, which is heated slowly until the milk solids precipitate out, or by the traditional (*desi*) method, in which fresh, unhomogenized milk is turned into yogurt (*dahi*), which is then mixed with water and churned. The cream comes out on top, and is then heated like butter until the milk solids precipitate out. The latter method produces almost twice as much con-

jugated linoleic acid as t[...]
1991), but is not used am[...]
brands of ghee. We give [...]
(using the former method [...]
practicable for most read[...]
chapter.

Milk

In addition to ghee, MAV and traditional Vedic texts also emphasize the healthfulness of cow's milk. According to Ayurveda, cow's milk rejuvenates, nourishes, and strengthens the body, promotes longevity, and soothes the mind. It balances all the *doshas*, and particularly reduces *Pitta*. It is considered sweet and astringent in taste, light in quality, and cooling. It is recommended especially for those who are weak or convalescent. (In Western terms, it is an excellent source of calcium, which makes it especially valuable for women in preventing osteoporosis; it is of course far better to get calcium from food than from supplements, which can interfere with nutrient assimilation.)

As with ghee, the view that milk is too fatty for cardiovascular health is not borne out by all research. The Maasai population of Kenya, who live on milk (4 liters per day), have low levels of cholesterol and a low incidence of cardiovascular mortality (Mann & Spoerry 1974, Gibney & Burstyn 1980). Also, in a clinical study published in the *Lancet*, drinking milk (4 pints per day for both males and females) significantly lowered the LDL cholesterol level, while the high-density lipoprotein (the 'good' cholesterol) level remained unchanged (Howard & Marks 1977).

A popular complaint against cow's milk is that it produces excess mucus. This is debatable (see Pinnock et al 1990, Pinnock & Arney 1993), but, when it occurs, MAV would suggest a factor rarely considered. Mucus is the waste product (*mala*) of *Kapha*; cold, oily foods aggravate or increase *Kapha*. Problems with milk, in this analysis, might result from its being taken cold. In fact, MAV traditionally has cautioned against drinking milk cold, because it is considered too hard to digest, and because it aggravates *Kapha*. It says that milk should always be boiled before drinking, not just to sterilize it, but to break down complex proteins and other compounds and make the milk easier to digest. To increase digestibility further, it also suggests

nch of ginger powder or fresh ginger to the
ile boiling.

AV also recommends not mixing milk with sour
salty foods, because they make the milk curdle
inside the stomach, which again makes the milk harder to digest, and also causes it to aggravate *Pitta*. It
should also not be taken at a full meal where mixed
tastes are served, though it can be taken with foods of
sweet taste, like toast or cereal.

Lactose intolerance, caused by insufficient production of the β-galactosidase enzyme, is common in certain populations, and its incidence increases with age
in many populations (Scientific Commission 1987).
The symptoms are easy to describe: a large glass of
milk brings on gas, diarrhea, and bloating, all caused
by the undigested milk sugar fermenting in the digestive tract; more precise measurements look at increases in breath hydrogen levels in the hours after
drinking milk. The condition is not absolute, but relative. People who had diagnosed themselves as lactose-
intolerant were shown to be able to digest a cup of
milk with no symptoms (Suarez et al 1995). For larger
amounts of milk, or if the intolerance is extreme, milk
in which the lactose has been predigested is now sold
commercially, and tablets of the lactase enzyme are
also available. Also, those with this condition often
have no problem with yogurt if it contains certain live
cultures (Gilliland & Kim 1984, Kolars et al 1984, Lin
et al 1991, Wytock & DiPalma 1988). This ability is lost
if the yogurt is heated before serving or (in most cases)
if it is frozen. For this reason, an excellent source of
milk nutrients for those intolerant of lactose is the
yogurt-based beverage called *lassi*, which is described
in the next section.

Yogurt and Ayurvedic 'buttermilk'

Yogurt is said to increase appetite and strength. It
increases *Kapha*, reduces *Vata*, and aggravates *Pitta*.
Yogurt is hot in quality and sour in taste (after it is
digested, though, its effect is like that of sweet foods).
It would be contraindicated, in fact, for those with
Pitta problems, especially in the digestive system:
those with ulcers, for example, should not use yogurt,
or for that matter, cheese. Milk, however, is excellent
for them.

Yogurt and cheese should not be taken at night,

because they tend to clog the channels of the body
when they are not digested well. Yogurt should
always be sweetened or taken with other foods, rather
than taken plain and alone.

It is best to make yogurt fresh (recipes are easy to
find), but if you buy commercially prepared yogurt,
try to get the most natural and fresh variety available.
Some brands try to keep the bacterial cultures in the
yogurt active and alive. These cultures benefit the
digestive tract. If commercial yogurt has been heated
after fermentation, though, the cultures are killed.
Also, some brands available in health-food stores use
organic and even non-homogenized milk; these are
preferable.

Ayurveda holds that the most beneficial way to take
yogurt, a way that very much improves its influence
on the *doshas'* balance, is in a beverage called
Ayurvedic buttermilk, which is not at all like commercial American buttermilk.

Buttermilk and lassi are beverages made of yogurt,
but have very different effects than does yogurt alone.
They are strengthening, and increase the appetite and
digestive power. They pacify all three *doshas*, and are
considered an excellent staple in anyone's diet. We
give a recipe for making them in Appendix 3 to this
chapter.

Why MAV recommends Lactovegetarianism

While vegetarianism is not required in order to benefit
from MAV, it is usually recommended, because for
most people it is a healthier diet. For one thing, meat
today usually has carcinogens and other chemicals
embedded in its excess fat cells, and fat is abundant no
matter how lean the cut. This brings us to the second
reason: even organically fed meat has high levels of
lipids; these lipids become peroxidized during digestion, and then interact with bile salts from the liver to
create disease-causing free radicals. The combination
of animal fat, bile acids, and bacterial flora in the colon
may produce carcinogens and cancer promoters.
Research has found long-term vegetarians to have
reduced risk of lipid peroxidation (Krajcovicova-
Kudlackova et al 1995a, 1995b).

Another advantage of a meatless diet is that it is
lighter and easier to digest, and, as we have seen, in

MAV ease of digestion is considered extremely important. Meat is difficult to digest because it has so many long-chain fatty acids, which are not completely metabolized by the body.

The American Cancer Society recommends reduced meat consumption to help reduce the risk of digestive-tract cancer. An excellent review by Dwyer (1988) covered hundreds of medical studies on vegetarianism, and found that the evidence was 'fair to good' for a lower incidence of diabetes mellitus mortality (about half that of meat-eaters), coronary artery disease mortality, gallstones, and hypertension. The evidence was 'good to excellent' for lower incidence of lung cancer, atonic constipation, and obesity. A number of studies have been published since then; their findings suggest that vegetarians have a significantly lower incidence of coronary heart disease (Slattery et al 1991, Claude-Chang et al 1992), and that vegetarianism can actively help reduce coronary heart disease (Ornish et al 1990). Another study found that women who eat red meat daily are at twice the risk of developing colon cancer than women who eat red meat less than once a month (Willett et al 1990). A long-term study of Seventh-Day Adventists found that, among males, meat-eating correlated with all forms of mortality measured (Snowdon 1988).

The fear that vegetarianism must necessarily lead to malnutrition has been shown to be unfounded; it depends on the type of vegetarian diet. Vegan diets, which exclude any animal products, have serious risks in this respect (Dwyer 1988), especially for children, but the lactovegetarianism recommended by MAV does not if it is balanced.

EATING TO CREATE HEALTH

When we eat, we participate in the creative processes of nature – the processes which create us again and again. Every 5 weeks, we get a new set of cells for our stomach lining; every month a new skin. Food provides the material for these overhauls. But according to MAV, it does more: *how* we eat determines how perfect the overhaul will be. If we feel emotionally ragged when we eat, food may disrupt rather than sustain the body's order. If we eat too quickly or overeat, the poorly digested end-products will predispose us to disease, not to health.

The advice given in this chapter is mea[...] food to contribute order and coherence to th[...] the body that MAV looks upon as a dynamic p[...] of knowledge more than a collection of matter. It a[...] helps the body keep balance, which is the essence of maintaining immune strength.

In the next chapter we focus on a more specific form of ingested substance, herbal mixtures that play a central role in MAV preventive and treatment programs.

APPENDIX 1. DIETS TO PACIFY *KAPHA*, *PITTA*, AND *VATA*

THE *KAPHA*-PACIFYING DIET SIMPLIFIED

Favor foods that are:
- Light
- Dry
- Warm
- Spicy
- Bitter (e.g. green leafy vegetables)
- Astringent (e.g. beans)

Reduce foods that are:
- Heavy
- Oily
- Cold
- Sweet (e.g. sugar, wheat)
- Salty (e.g. potato chips)
- Sour (e.g. sour citrus, cheese, yogurt)

Some specific recommendations for the *Kapha* diet

1. *Dairy*. Reduced use of milk is better for *Kaphas*. It is better to boil milk before drinking it (which makes it easier to digest), and it should always be taken warm in any case. It should not be taken with meals that include all six tastes (it mixes well with the sweet taste only), especially sour or salty foods. If one tends towards *Kapha* disorders like congestion, one might add one or two pinches of turmeric or ginger to milk before boiling it, to help reduce its *Kapha*-increasing qualities. Also, low-fat milk is preferable.

Avoid yogurt, cream, ice cream, cheese, butter, or large quantities of whole milk.

2. *Fruit*. Lighter, more astringent fruits like apples, pears, cranberries, persimmons, and pomegranates are better. Reduce heavy, very sweet, or sour fruits, like grapes, oranges, bananas, pineapple, figs, dates, avocados, coconuts, and melons, all of which increase *Kapha*.

h has an astringent quali-
...ha. It should be used in
...however, increase *Kapha*.
... nuts.

... Barley, millet, corn, rye,
... *Kaphas*, but use of wheat,
oats, and rice, which ...rease *Kapha dosha*, should
be reduced.

6. *Spices*. All are suitable, except for salt, which
increases *Kapha*.

7. *Vegetables*. All are fine, except for tomatoes,
cucumbers, okra, sweet potatoes, and zucchini.

8. *Oils*. *Kaphas* should avoid large amounts of any
oil; small amounts of almond and sesame oil are fine.

9. *Meat and fish*. Meat is not recommended, but
those patients who cannot do without should eat the
white meat from chicken and turkey. Avoid red meat
(e.g. beef, veal, and pork), however, and most seafood.

THE *PITTA*-PACIFYING DIET SIMPLIFIED

Favor foods that are:
- Cold
- Heavy
- Oily
- Sweet (e.g. wheat. milk, rice)
- Bitter
- Astringent

Reduce foods that are:
- Warm
- Light
- Dry
- Spicy
- Salty
- Sour (e.g. tomatoes, cheese, yogurt, citrus)

Some specific recommendations for the *Pitta* diet

1. *Dairy*. Milk, butter, and ghee are good for pacifying *Pitta*. Reduce use of yogurt, cheese, sour cream,
and cultured buttermilk, for their sour tastes aggravate *Pitta*.

2. *Sweeteners*. All sweeteners are good for *Pitta*
except for honey and molasses in large quantities.

3. *Oils*. Besides butter and ghee, olive and coconut
oils are the best. *Pittas* should reduce the use of sesame,
almond, and corn oil, all of which increase *Pitta*.

4. *Grains*. Wheat, white rice, barley, and oats are
good. Reduce corn, millet, rye, and brown rice.

5. *Fruits*. Favor sweet fruits, such as grapes, cherries,
melons, avocado, coconut, pomegranate, mangos, and
sweet oranges, pineapples, and plums. Reduce sour
fruits, such as grapefruit, olives, underripe pineapples
or persimmons, sour or unripe oranges, unripe bananas,
and some plums.

6. *Vegetables*. Favor asparagus, pumpkin, carrots,
cucumber, cabbage, potato, sweet potato, okra, green
beans, green leafy vegetables, broccoli, cauliflower,
celery, sprouts, zucchini. Avoid hot peppers, radish,
tomatoes, beets, onions, and garlic.

7. *Beans*. Only lentils, mung beans, and tofu are
good for *Pitta*.

8. *Spices*. Fennel, cinnamon, turmeric, coriander, and
cardamom are suitable. *Small* amounts of ginger, cumin,
and black pepper are fine. The following spices increase
Pitta, so they too should be used only in small amounts:
cloves, celery seed, fenugreek, salt, and mustard seed.
Avoid cayenne and chilis, which aggravate *Pitta*.

9. *Meats*. Chicken, pheasant, and turkey are acceptable; but red meat, seafood, and egg yolk increase *Pitta*
(though egg whites do not).

THE *VATA*-PACIFYING DIET SIMPLIFIED

Note: This diet may be too heavy for *Vatas* if their
digestion is irregular or weak. If this applies, see the
section below on the 'purifying diet'.

Favor foods that are:
- Warm
- Oily
- Heavy
- Sweet (e.g. wheat, milk, rice)
- Sour (e.g. yogurt, tomatoes, citrus fruit)
- Salty

Reduce foods that are:
- Cold
- Dry
- Light
- Spicy
- Bitter (e.g. green leafy vegetables)
- Astringent (e.g. apples, beans)

Some specific recommendations for the *Vata* diet

1. Eat larger quantities of food, but not more than
can be digested easily.

2. *Dairy*. All dairy products pacify *Vata*. It is better
to boil milk before drinking it (for ease of digestion),
and to drink it warm. Do not take milk with a full meal
that includes many tastes; milk mixes well only with
the sweet taste, e.g. toast or breakfast cereal.

3. *Sweeteners*. Raw sugar, brown sugar, molasses,

and honey are good for *Vata* if taken in reasonable amounts.

4. *Oils*. All oils reduce *Vata*.

5. *Grains*. Rice and wheat are very good. Reduce intake of barley, corn, millet, buckwheat, rye, oats.

6. *Fruits*. Favor sweet, sour, or heavy fruits, such as oranges, bananas, avocados, grapes, cherries, peaches, melons, berries, plums, fresh figs, sweet pineapples, mangos and papayas. Take fewer dry, light, or astringent fruits, such as apples, pears, pomegranates, cranberries, and dried fruits.

7. *Vegetables*. Beets, carrots, asparagus, cucumbers, and sweet potatoes are good. They should be cooked, not raw. The following vegetables are *acceptable* in moderate quantities if they are cooked, and also if they are then moistened with a little ghee, vegetable oil, or butter and flavored with a small amount of *Vata*-reducing spices: peas, green leafy vegetables, broccoli, cauliflower, celery, zucchini, green beans, potatoes. It is better to avoid sprouts and cabbage salads and all raw vegetables.

8. *Spices*. Cardamom, cumin, ginger, cinnamon, salt, cloves, mustard seed, and small quantities of black pepper are suitable. Minimize red peppers and chilis.

9. All *nuts* are good.

10. Reduce intake of *beans*, all of which increase *Vata*, except for tofu and mung dahl. (Note: this does not refer to green beans, which are a vegetable.)

11. *Meats*. Chicken, turkey and seafoods are acceptable for non-vegetarians; rabbit, pheasant, and red meat should be avoided. (You may have noticed that red meat is not recommended in any of the diets. This ancient Ayurvedic advice presages the modern medical view that one should limit one's intake of red meat.)

IMPORTANT NOTE

These diets will not apply to all individuals. For example, those with a known or suspected problem with high blood lipids (e.g. cholesterol) should consult their physician before increasing fats or oils in their diet.

APPENDIX 2. HOW TO MAKE GHEE

Having described above the benefits of ghee, we include here a recipe for preparing it. The preferred way, as explained, is to use the cream from yogurt made of non-homogenized milk. Since that is very hard to procure, we include below the recipe for making ghee from unsalted butter.

SET-UP

You will need:

- A 1.5 or 2 quart pot, preferably glass, enameled, or stainless steel (copper or iron pots will leave metallic impurities in the ghee which shorten its shelf-life).
- A stove or burner with a rheostat.
- A stainless steel or silver spoon.
- 1 lb of unsalted butter (salted will work, but not as well).
- A meat thermometer (optional).
- A perfectly dry 1-pint container to put the finished ghee in; ceramic or glass is best, but don't use a rubber seal, as the rubber tends to dissolve into the ghee.
- A filter made of clean, fine-weave, white cloth, or a 2-foot square cheesecloth. (Alternatively, you can use a coffee filter system with paper filters; this is not ideal unless you clean it thoroughly with baking soda, detergent and hot water to remove all the coffee flavor.)
- A work surface impervious to oil.
- $1\frac{1}{2}$ hours of your time. *Important:* Do not leave the ghee unattended at any time in the cooking process; any oil can burn when overheated.

COOKING THE GHEE

1. Melt the butter in the pot, which is left uncovered (the water in the butter must boil away). Use the 'medium' or 'medium-low' setting on your burner. (A higher heat will speed up the process but often scorches the ghee.)

2. In 3 to 5 minutes, the butter will melt. From this point on, be careful not to let it scorch. As soon as it bubbles or begins to boil, turn the heat down to low and let it simmer. Tiny bubbles will be forming at the bottom and occasionally rising to the top.

3. After about 20 minutes, the temperature of the

ghee will reach about 212°F, the boiling point of water, and will remain there while the water is boiling out (30 to 40 minutes).

While this long, slow simmer is going on, the milk solids, which look white and foamy, are separating out. Some will sink to the bottom, others will float. Stir the ghee a few times during this stage and take the spoon and gently push to the sides any solids that are floating (i.e. that have not sunk to the bottom).

4. Be alert to when all the water has boiled out so that you can quickly remove the ghee pan from the heat to avoid scorching the liquid. If you have a thermometer, you will notice that when the water is gone the temperature will rise quickly – turn the heat off when the ghee reaches 240°F. Other indications that the ghee is done are that: the heavy boiling (water) sounds change to the light sizzle of bubbles rising from the bottom; the ghee has a rich aroma similar to popcorn; and the milk solids at the bottom of the pan turn golden brown. As soon as you notice these signs, turn off the heat.

5. Strain the sediment from the ghee while hot. For optimum results, pour through a folded cheesecloth or cotton cloth into a clean, dry glass or ceramic container. Make the cloth dip down into the jar about 1″ and secure it with a rubber band around the jar's mouth. The cloth can also be laid over a stainless steel strainer placed over the jar's mouth. Since the ghee is very hot, be careful as you pour it. Scrape the sides and bottom of the pan with a spoon so that all the solids go into the filter. Do not push the solids through the filter – let solids drain for about 2 to 3 minutes, then discard them when you remove the filter.

6. Let the ghee cool at room temperature until the container is cool to the touch. Then cover it and store at room temperature; there is no need to refrigerate it. Ghee liquifies when warm and solidifies when cooler.

APPENDIX 3. HOW TO MAKE AYURVEDIC 'BUTTERMILK' AND LASSI

The ideal way to make 'buttermilk' and lassi is to make fresh yogurt using non-homogenized milk, which, admittedly, is not always easy to obtain; the milk can be pasteurized, however, as long as it is non-homogenized. Some commercially available brands of yogurt are made of non-homogenized milk and can be used for this recipe. After you have made (or bought) the yogurt, mix it with an equal part of water in the blender (don't use hot water, which would kill the bacterial cultures) at a low speed – as if you were churning cream. After 1–2 minutes the fat in the yogurt will separate out and rise to the top; this should be skimmed off. What is left is what Ayurveda calls 'buttermilk'. It is considered an ideal beverage, which can be taken at every meal if desired. You may add some ginger, cumin, or other spices, or sweeteners, depending on the season and your body type. If *Vata* is aggravated, you can add a little salt or sweetener, and some cumin; if *Pitta* needs reducing, you can use raw or brown sugar; if *Kapha*, add ginger, black pepper and a little honey.

Because non-homogenized milk or yogurt may be hard to get, many people use a substitute recipe. Take one part non-fat yogurt, three parts water, and mix well in a blender. You may flavor it as above. This is called lassi. It is considered to be less beneficial than Ayurvedic buttermilk, but still an excellent staple.

REFERENCES

Aneja R P, Murthi T N 1991 Beneficial effects of ghee. Nature 350:280

Beilin L J 1987 Diet and hypertension: critical concepts and controversies. Journal of Hypertension 5 (Suppl 5):S447–S457

Claude-Chang J, Frentzel-Beyme R, Eilber U 1992 Mortality pattern of German vegetarians after 11 years of follow-up. Epidemiology 3(5):395–401

Crosser A E, Mistry V V, Sharma H M, Dwivedi C 1994 Effects of butter oil, ghee, corn oil, or safflower oil on blood cholesterol, triglycerides and lipoprotein in rats. Paper presented at the Annual Meeting of Dairy Science, Minneapolis, Minn, July 1994

Darlington L G, Ramsey N W, Mansfield J R 1986 Placebo controlled, blind study of dietary manipulation therapy in rheumatoid arthritis. Lancet 1:236–238

Dwyer J T 1988 Health aspects of vegetarian diets. American Journal of Clinical Nutrition 48:712–38

Gibney M J, Burstyn P G 1980 Milk, serum cholesterol, and the Maasai. Atherosclerosis 35:339–343

Gilliland S E, Kim H S 1984 Effect of viable starter culture bacteria in yogurt on lactose utilization in humans. Journal of Dairy Science 67:1–9

Hafstrom I, Ringertz B, Gyllenhammer H 1988 Effects of fasting on disease activity, neutrophil function, fatty acids composition, and leukotriene biosynthesis in patients with rheumatoid arthritis. Arthritis and Rheumatism 31(5):585–592

Hageman G, Verhagen H, Schutte B, Kleinjans J 1991 Biological effects of short-term feeding to rats of repeatedly used deep-frying fats in relation to fat mutagen content. Food Chemical Toxicology 29:689–698

Hicklin J A, McEwen L M, Morgan J E 1989 The effect of diet on rheumatoid arthritis. Clinical Allergy 10:463–467

Hills B A 1990 Physical identity for the gastric mucosal barrier. Medical Journal of Australia 153:76–81

Howard A N, Marks J 1977 Hypocholesterolaemic effect of milk. Lancet 2:255–256

Jacobson M S 1987 Cholesterol oxides in Indian ghee. Lancet 2:656–658

Kolars J C, Levitt M D, Aouji M, Saviano D A 1984 Yogurt – an autodigesting source of lactose. New England Journal of Medicine 310(1):1–3

Krajcovicova-Kudlackova M, Simoncic R, Bederova A, Klvanova J, Babinska K, Granciconva E 1995a Plasma fatty acid profile and prooxidative-antioxidative parameters in vegetarians. Nahrung 39(5–6):452–457

Krajcovicova-Kudlackova M, Simoncic R, Babinska K, Bederova A 1995b Levels of lipid peroxidation and anti-oxidants in vegetarians. European Journal of Epidemiology 11(2):207–211

Lin M Y, Savaiano D, Harlander S 1991 Influence of non-fermented dairy products containing bacterial starter cultures on lactose maldigestion in humans. Journal of Dairy Science 74:87–95

Mann G V, Spoerry A 1974 Studies of a surfactant and cholesteremia in the Masai. American Journal of Clinical Nutrition 27:464–469

Mensink R P M, Katan M B 1990 Effects of dietary trans fatty acids on high-density and low-density lipoprotein cholesterol levels in healthy subjects. New England Journal of Medicine 323:439–445

Nath B S, Rama Murthy M K 1988 Cholesterol in Indian ghee. Lancet 2:39

Ornish D, Brown S E, Scherwitz L W et al 1990 Can lifestyle changes reverse coronary heart disease? The Lifestyle Heart Trial. Lancet 336:129–133

Pinnock C B, Arney W K 1993 The milk-mucus belief: sensory analysis comparing cow's milk and a soy placebo. Appetite 20(1):61–70

Pinnock C B, Graham N M, Mylvaganam A, Douglas R M 1990 Relationship between milk intake and mucus production in adult volunteers challenged with rhinovirus-2. American Review of Respiratory Disease 141(2):352–356

Profet M 1992 Pregnancy sickness as adaptation: a deterrent to maternal ingestion of teratogens. In: Barkow J H, Cosmides L, Tooby J (eds) The adapted mind. Oxford University Press, New York, pp. 327–366

Schrödinger E 1967 What is life? Cambridge University Press, Cambridge

Scientific Commission for Nutritional Research on Fresh Milk Products 1987 A critical analysis of the major French and foreign studies on yoghurt. In: Yogurt and its live bacteria. (SEPAIC, Paris, Cahiers de nutrition diététique, p 12)

Sharma H 1990 Butter oil (ghee) – myths and facts. Indian Journal of Clinical Practice 1(2):31–32

Skoldstam L, Larsson L, Linstrom F 1979 Effects of fasting and lactovegetarian diet on rheumatoid arthritis. Scandanavian Journal of Rheumatology 2:249–255

Slattery M, Jacobs O R Jr, Hilner J E et al 1991 Meat consumption and its associations with other diet and health factors in young adults: the CARDIA study. American Journal of Clinical Nutrition 54:930–935

Snowdon D A 1988 Animal product consumption and mortality because of all causes combined, coronary heart disease, stroke, diabetes, and cancer in Seventh-Day Adventists. American Journal of Clinical Nutrition 58:739–748

Stroud R M 1983 The effect of fasting followed by specific food challenge on rheumatoid arthritis. In: Kahn B H, Arnett F, Zizix T, Hochberg M (eds) Current topics in rheumatology. Upjohn, Kalamazoo

Suarez F L, Savaiano D A, Levitt M D 1995 A comparison of symptoms after the consumption of milk or lactose-hydrolyzed milk by people with self-reported severe lactose intolerance. New England Journal of Medicine 333(1):1–4

Uden A M, Trang L, Venizeloz N, Palmblad J 1983 Neutrophil function and clinical performance after total fasting in patients with rheumatoid arthritis. Ann Rheum Dis 42:45–51

Willett W C, Ascherio A 1994 Trans fatty acids: are the effects only marginal? American Journal of Public Health 84:722–724

Willet W C, Stampfer M J, Colditz G A, Rosner B A, Speizer F E 1990 Relation of meat, fat and fiber intake to the risk of colon cancer in a prospective study among women. New England Journal of Medicine 323: 1664–1672

Wurtman T J, Wurtman R J, Growden J 1981 Carbohydrate craving in obese people. International Journal of Eating Disorders 1:2–15

Wurtman T J, Wurtman R J, Mark S 1985 D-fenfluramine selectively suppresses carbohydrate snacking by obese subjects. International Journal of Eating Disorders 4:89–99

Wytock D H, DiPalma J A 1988 All yogurts are not created equal. American Journal of Clinical Nutrition 47:454–457

8

Active ingredients, free radicals, and the herbal pharmacopeia

Like humans, plants need to protect themselves against toxins and pathogens, which come from both within and without. Like human bodies, plants produce chemicals for that purpose. Not surprisingly, these chemicals can benefit human bodies as well – a fact well-known to both Western and Ayurvedic pharmacology. Ayurvedic pharmacology (called *dravyaguna*) differs from modern pharmacology in a crucial way. *Dravyaguna* uses plants (or plant parts) as they occur in nature, with all their ingredients. Western pharmacology – which applies a 'machine' model of the body – isolates active ingredients from plants, then (usually) synthesizes them.

The majority of Western medications have been derived, in this way, from natural substances. For example, Western researchers derived acetylsalicylic acid from the pain remedy willow bark, and the antihypertensive/antipsychotic drug reserpine from *Rauwolfia serpentina*, a herb prescribed in ancient Ayurvedic texts for mental disorders. Medical science tends to assume that the replacement of natural herbs with synthetic active ingredients is an unambiguous leap of progress.

However, the active ingredient approach compromises whatever synergies exist among organic components, which can be significant. Also, many apparently inactive ingredients have turned out to play significant health-giving roles. For example, the medical value of bioflavonoids (a class of molecules found in plants) was often dismissed by early researchers, especially those who favored artificial vitamins, which they saw as the plants' active ingredients. But many bioflavonoids have since been found to have significant benefits. They act as antioxidant, anti-inflammatory, anti-allergic, antitumor, anti-ulcerogenic, and hepatoprotective agents. Who knows what other valuable compounds remain, as yet unidentified, in plants?

Finally, the active ingredient approach relates to the issue of side-effects. Western pharmaceuticals frequently create unwanted side-effects, sometimes serious. Active ingredients act indiscriminately, not only at the site intended but also at other sites and organs; this is why toxicity arises. With whole herbs, inactive ingredients are thought to help control the effects at non-target sites.

To illustrate the limitations of the active-ingredient approach in distinction to herbal pharmacology, we review the research that has emerged on certain herbal formulations, and their effect on free radical formation.

HERBAL FORMULATIONS AS ANTIOXIDANTS

To understand the implications of the research on the herbal formulas, we begin our discussion by examining a recent development in medical theory.

A decade ago it might have seemed absurd to suggest that cataracts, rheumatoid arthritis, and strokes may all have one basic source of damage in common, or that the etiology of cancer, heart disease, and dandruff may share a common mechanism. But now the evidence for this unified understanding is growing. For much of aging and disease a common link in the causal chain is molecules known as free radicals.

Many regard discovery of the medical role of free radicals as being as big an advance as Pasteur's theory of infectious disease. In a sense, free radicals take medical theory one step deeper. Pasteur's discovery involved microorganisms and cells; free radicals involve a more fundamental level – the subatomic realm of electrons.

Free radicals, as we mentioned briefly in Chapter 3, are molecules, usually of oxygen, that have lost an electron. This makes them unstable (in chemical terms, *reactive*). They begin to powerfully covet their neighboring molecules' electrons. In stealing an electron, they can become terrorists in our bodies. They can attack DNA, leading to dysfunction, mutation, and cancer. They can attack enzymes and proteins, disrupting normal cell activities. They can attack cell membranes, producing a chain reaction of destruction. Such membrane damage

in the cells that line our blood vessels can lead to hardening and thickening of the arteries and eventually to heart attacks and strokes. Free radical attacks on the protein in collagen can cause cross-linking of protein molecules and resulting stiffness in the tissue.

The most dangerous free radicals are the small, mobile, and highly reactive oxy radicals. Other dangerous atomic and molecular varieties of oxygen are known as reactive oxygen species (ROS). These are not technically free radicals, but they are none the less unstable and highly reactive with the molecules around them. Increasing biomedical research is demonstrating that oxidative stress – the constant attack by oxy radicals and reactive oxygen species – is important in both the initiation and promotion stages of many major diseases. They help cause the disease in the first place, then add impetus to its spread in the body. In the case of heart disease, oxidative stress can cause major damage even after treatment has been applied.

The implications go further. It now appears that the 'clinical presentation' of different diseases – the way the illness appears when a patient comes to the clinic – may be due not to different causal mechanisms, but to variations in the protection provided by the body's antioxidant defenses. In a hurricane, the weakest link in a house will go – whether doors or windows or an insecure roof. Under oxidative stress, the weakest link in the body may give way.

The list of diseases now linked to oxy radicals and reactive oxygen species (ROS) is long and disturbing (Box 8.1).

The onslaught of free radicals and ROS also contributes to many of the less serious but still troubling symptoms of aging: not only wrinkled and unresilient skin, but also gray hair, balding, and bodily stiffness. Oxy radicals and ROS have been linked to such minor but bothersome conditions like dandruff and hangovers. One of the most experienced researchers in the field, the Japanese biochemist Yukie Niwa, estimates that at least 85% of chronic and degenerative diseases are the result of oxidative damage (Niwa & Hansen 1989, p 9).

BENEFITS OF FREE RADICALS

Despite the lengthy list of problems they cause, free radicals are not all bad. They have vital roles to play in

---

Box 8.1   Diseases linked to oxy radicals and reactive oxygen species

- Cancer.
- Arteriosclerosis, atherosclerosis.
- Heart disease.
- Cerebrovascular disease.
- Stroke.
- Emphysema (Cross et al 1987).
- Diabetes mellitus (Sato et al 1979).
- Rheumatoid arthritis (Cross et al 1987, Greenwald & Moy 1979, 1980, Halliwell 1981, 1989, Del Maestro et al 1982, Fligiel et al 1984).
- Osteoporosis (Hooper 1989, Stringer et al 1989).
- Ulcers.
- Sunburn.
- Cataracts (Niwa & Hansen 1989, Yagi 1977).
- Crohn's disease (Niwa & Hansen 1989)
- Behçet's disease.
- Senility.
- Aging.

---

a healthy human body. In the first place, certain types of free radicals are inevitably produced by many chemical reactions that occur in the body. The body can, however, usually keep control over the free radicals that typically result. Second, the body attempts to harness the destructive power of the most dangerous free radicals – the small and highly reactive oxy radicals and ROS – for use in the immune system and inflammatory reactions. Certain cells in these systems engulf bacteria or viruses, taking up oxygen molecules from the bloodstream, creating a flood of oxy radicals and ROS by removing an electron, and bombarding the invader with this toxic shower. To an impressive degree, this aggressive use of toxic oxygen species succeeds in protecting the body against infectious organisms.

Unfortunately, the process may go out of control, creating a destructive chain reaction that leads to overproduction of free radicals. Like other formations of free radicals, this can wreak havoc in the body.

THE CAUSES OF FREE RADICALS

Production of free radicals in the body is continuous and inescapable. The basic causes are:

Energy production

The energy-producing process in every cell generates oxy radicals and ROS as toxic waste, continuously and in abundance. Oxygen is used to burn glucose molecules that act as the body's fuel. In this energy-freeing operation, oxy radicals are thrown off as destructive by-products. Given the insatiable electron hunger of oxygen, there is no way to have it suffusing the body's energy-producing processes without the constant creation of oxy radicals and ROS.

The cell has a complex structure and function, including a number of metabolic processes. Each of these can produce different free radicals. Thus, even a single cell can produce many different kinds of free radicals.

Immune system

As we have just seen, immune system cells create oxy radicals and ROS deliberately, as weapons.

Pollution and other external substances

In modern life, we are constantly exposed to external substances that generate free radicals in the body. The food most of us buy contains farm chemicals, including fertilizers and pesticides, that, when we ingest the food, produce free radicals as by-products. The same is true for many prescription drugs; their harmful side-effects may be caused by the free radicals they generate. Processed foods frequently contain high levels of lipid peroxides, which produce free radicals that damage the cardiovascular system. Cigarette smoke generates high free radical concentrations; much lung damage associated with smoking is caused by free radicals. The same is true of environmental pollution. Alcohol is a particularly potent free radical generator. In addition, all types of electromagnetic radiation can cause free radicals – including, unfortunately, sunlight. When sunlight hits the skin, it generates free radicals which then age the skin, causing roughness and wrinkles. If the exposure is severe and prolonged, skin cancer may be one result (Box 8.2).

Stress

The fast pace of modern life is also a recipe for free radicals. The constant pressure and time-shortage

---

Box 8.2 Some common external causes of free radicals

- Toxins
  - carbon tetrachloride
  - paraquat
  - benzo(a)pyrene
  - aniline dyes
  - Toluene

- Drugs
  - adriamycin
  - bleomycin
  - mitomycin C
  - nitrofurantoin
  - chlorpromazine

- Air pollution
  Primary sources
  - carbon monoxide
  - nitric oxide
  - unburned hydrocarbons
  Secondary sources
  - ozone
  - nitrogen dioxide
  - aldehydes
  - alkyl nitrates

- Radiation, sunlight
- Ingested substances
  - Alcohol
  - Tobacco smoke
  - Smoked and barbecued food
  - Peroxidized fats in meat and cheese
  - Deep-fried foods

---

experienced by most people in industrialized countries causes them to experience high levels of stress. And the stress response in the body creates free radicals in abundance. It races the body's energy-creating apparatus, increasing the number of free radicals created as toxic waste. Moreover, the hormones which mediate the stress reaction in the body – cortisol and catecholamines – themselves degenerate into particularly destructive free radicals. Researchers now know one way in which stress may cause disease. A stressful life mass-produces free radicals.

FREE RADICAL DEFENSES

Given the many sources of free radicals, all aerobic forms of life maintain elaborate anti-free-radical defense systems (also known as antioxidant systems).

Enzymes

Every cell in the body creates its own 'bomb squad' – antioxidant enzymes (complex, machine-like proteins) whose particular job it is to defuse oxy radicals and ROS. One of the most destructive free radicals, for example, is superoxide. The most thoroughly studied defense enzyme, known as superoxide dismutase (SOD), takes hold of superoxide molecules and changes them to a much less reactive form.

SOD and other important antioxidant enzymes, the glutathione system, work within the cell. By contrast, circulating biochemicals such as uric acid and cerulo-

plasmin react with free radicals in the intercellular spaces and bloodstream.

Nutrients

As a second tier, the body makes use of many standard vitamins and other nutrients, including vitamins C, E, beta-carotene, bioflavonoids, and many others, to quench the oxy radicals' thirst for electrons. Many free radical researchers feel that to quench free radicals effectively the general levels of all these free radical-fighting nutrients need to be much higher than nutritional experts previously thought. (This demonstrates how the substances that plants create to fight free radicals can help the human body do the same thing.)

Self-repair

In addition to using enzymes and nutrients for direct attacks on oxy radicals, the body also has a rapid and thorough system to repair and/or replace damaged building blocks of the cell. For example, the system for repairing damage to DNA and other nucleic acids is particularly elaborate and efficient, involving separate specific enzymes which first locate damaged areas, then snip out ruined bits, replace them with the correct sequence of molecules, and seal up the strand once again. Every aspect of the cell is given similar attention. Most protein constituents in the cell, for example, are completely replaced every few days. Scavenger enzymes break used and damaged proteins into their component parts for reuse by the cell.

FINDING THE BALANCE

The body's elaborate biochemical responses to the free radical challenge suggest that it is not necessary to reduce excess free radicals to zero. The body need only strike a proper balance between the number of free radicals generated and the defense and repair mechanisms available. The goal is to keep oxidative stress below the level at which normal repair and replacement can maintain 100% cell efficacy. Oxy radicals might slip through the enzyme and nutrient defenses to attack the DNA, for instance. But ideally these attacks would be few enough that the DNA repair mechanisms could fix the damage and maintain the genetic code intact.

How, then, can we keep that balance? This is a major topic of research; the results of the above approaches have been mixed. Vitamins and beta-carotene have shown far fewer benefits than many expected. One long-term, large-scale study found beta-carotene to have no effect whatsoever in reducing malignant neoplasms, cardiovascular disease, or death from all causes (Hennekens et al 1996). One problem may be that active ingredients like beta-carotene are not 'full spectrum' antioxidants: they affect certain free radicals and not others (and each cell can produce a wide variety of free radicals). Two recent studies also suggest that there is another problem. Beta-carotene and vitamin E were found not to prevent lung cancer in male smokers; in fact, beta-carotene was linked with *higher* incidence of lung cancer (Alpha-Tocopherol, Beta Carotene Cancer Prevention Study Group 1994). Beta-carotene and vitamin A supplements, too, were found to increase risk of lung cancer in smokers and workers exposed to asbestos (Omenn et al 1996), and to have no offsetting benefits of any kind. A reason for the harmful effects may be that the vitamins, after quenching free radicals, become oxidized themselves unless they have been given in correct doses or regenerated by additional antioxidants, which must be in proper doses themselves. (Beta-carotene, moreover, works as an antioxidant only when oxygen concentrations are low; in high oxygen concentrations, such as those found in the lungs or heart, it becomes an oxidant itself (Burton & Ingold

1984). In addition, large amounts of any one micronutrient may inhibit absorption of other micronutrients needed for proper nutritional balance.

Such problems might be offset if vitamins were taken in their natural condition, surrounded by dozens of apparently inactive ingredients that modulate their effects. This conclusion is suggested by a study that found vitamin E to have no effect in reducing death from coronary heart disease in postmenopausal women when taken in the form of supplements, but to have significant benefits when absorbed from food (Kushi et al 1996).

Even if these problems with vitamin supplements were solved, a formidable one remains: the body's natural enzymes are, molecule for molecule, much more effective. When a molecule of vitamin C or E sacrifices an electron to appease a free radical, the vitamin molecule becomes damaged and useless. Only if it is regenerated by a helpful companion can it re-enter the fray. Enzymes, however, can run through thousands of destructive free radicals and ROS without help and without pause.

Yet although internally produced enzymes are far more powerful than vitamins, they cannot be taken by mouth. They are gigantic protein molecules that cannot pass through the walls of the digestive system and into the bloodstream. Digestive juices break them down into their component amino acids. Although SOD has been given by injection directly into inflamed joints, this is not practical for all-purpose home use. This is particularly so because SOD has only a brief half-life in the bloodstream: in less than 5 minutes, 50% of it is gone, broken down by natural bodily processes, and within an hour only 0.1% of it is left. Recently, the Japanese researcher Tatsuya Oda found a way around this: he succeeded in attaching SOD to artificial polymer molecules. Riding on the polymers, the SOD lasts in the bloodstream for at least 5 hours. But this raises questions about the long-term effects of adding an enzyme to the body in large quantities; these are not known as yet, and the question is far from trivial.

In an ideal world, we would find antioxidant substances with (1) low molecular weight, so they can slip from the digestive tract to the bloodstream undamaged, (2) the anti-free-radical ability, weight for weight, of an enzyme like SOD, and (3) the ability to defuse a wide range of free radicals. It may sound too much to hope for. But, if found, such powerful antioxidants might tip the scales against free radical damage decisively.

RASAYANAS

Powerful free radical scavengers that appear to fulfil the above criteria have been identified. These natural antioxidants scavenge superoxide as effectively as SOD. Weight for weight, they stop lipid peroxide chain reactions hundreds and even thousands of times better than antioxidant vitamins and a much-researched antioxidant drug. They are not active ingredients, like vitamin pills, but food supplements, and can be eaten and digested easily. As shown below, they combine natural plant products to create synergies, rather than isolating active ingredients.

Ayurvedic substances called *rasayanas* are herbal formulations that stimulate overall health. The term literally means 'that which supports *rasa*'. *Rasa*, as we've seen, is the first of the seven *dhatus*; it is equivalent to chyle and blood plasma, and is said to nourish all the other bodily tissues. *Rasayanas* are also said to stimulate the production of *ojas*, the substance that sustains all the *dhatus*.

Rasayanas can be useful in treating specific illnesses, but most of them are intended to increase general immune strength (known in Ayurveda as *bala* or life force) and general health and well-being. *Rasayanas* are held to promote general health by increasing resistance to disease, activating tissue repair mechanisms, and arresting or reversing the deterioration associated with aging. According to Charaka, *rasayanas* promote 'longevity, memory, intelligence, freedom from disorders, youthfulness, excellence of luster, complexion and voice, optimum strength of physique and sense organs...'

Such claims can be seen to fit with what research has shown about *rasayanas* and their effects on free radicals. According to many studies, the most effective response to the challenge of free radicals comes from one of the world's oldest systems of natural health care.

AN ANCIENT DISCOVERY

For all the promise of the research findings, *rasayanas* can make experts in Western medical science uneasy,

since they are not artificial drugs isolated in a test tube, but natural herbal mixtures from India's Vedic tradition that contain a rich variety of plant substances.

The recipes for these herbal formulations were first discovered thousands of years ago. As with much else in the ancient Vedic tradition, over the course of time knowledge of these herbal supplements was lost to the general public. The herbal formulas were carefully maintained, however, guarded and handed down through generations by a small number of Ayurvedic *vaidyas*.

In 1985, Maharishi Mahesh Yogi met with a number of the leading Ayurvedic *vaidyas* of our time, looking for additional knowledge from the Vedic tradition to make available to the modern world. Among the *vaidyas* present were Dr B. D. Triguna, then President of the All-India Ayurvedic Congress, and Director of the National Academy for Ayurveda, Government of India; the late Dr V. M. Dwivedi, Professor Emeritus, Gujarat Ayurvedic University, and former Vice-Chairman of the Indian Government's Ayurveda Pharmacopoeia Committee; and Dr Balraj Maharshi, an adviser on Ayurveda to the government of Andhra Pradesh, and perhaps the world's leading expert on *dravyaguna*, the identification and utilization of medicinal plants. Dr Dwivedi was one of the few remaining *vaidyas* in India who was a master of the procedures for creating *rasayanas*.

It was Dr Balraj Maharshi who first made a specific suggestion. Many years earlier he had studied with a venerable *vaidya* who had passed on to him the ancient formula for *amrit kalash* – with the admonition that it should only be revealed when the time had come it could be widely used. After saving the formula for many years, Dr Balraj Maharshi decided that *amrit kalash* now had the opportunity to be scientifically accepted. He shared the formula, and Maharishi asked him to work with Dr Triguna, Dr Dwivedi, and other *vaidyas* to restore the mixture and its preparation to the ancient standards recorded in the classical Ayurvedic texts. Dr Triguna, meanwhile, provided another ancient herbal formula of similar efficacy.

THE TRADITIONAL APPROACH TO PREPARATION

The results of this cooperative effort have been available in the West for about a decade. Maharishi Amrit Kalash (MAK) is in fact available in two separate formulations. One of these, MAK-4, is a herbal concentrate (from the formula provided by Dr Triguna); the other, MAK-5, is a herbal tablet (from the formula provided by Dr Balraj Maharshi). Between them they comprise more than 24 different herbs and fruits,* each of which is composed of hundreds of chemical substances – separate types of molecules.

Preparing the *rasayanas* involves subtleties unfamiliar to Western scientists. For example, plant chronobiology – choosing the optimum time to harvest a herb – is vital, since the presence and levels of phytochemicals (such as bioflavonoids) differ at different times of the year. Further, Ayurvedic herbs were traditionally prepared through a long and careful process of grinding. The goal was to reduce each component of a formula to the finest possible powder, and no effort was spared to reach this highly refined stage. Modern research suggests an explanation for this method of preparation. In a complex natural product, many of the important components are tangled together and unassimilable, and the grinding process apparently works to enhance their digestibility.

This whole process of formulation and preparation is an aspect of Maharishi Amrit Kalash that is disconcerting to Western scientists, who are used not to taking whole flowers, plants, and roots and grinding them down into an unanalyzable potpourri of various substances, but to seeking a single active ingredient, a 'magic bullet', to fire at each disease. They are also accustomed to the protocols of objective investigation – taking isolated substances made of identical molecules, testing them in the laboratory, putting them through human clinical trials, and finally prescribing them as cures for specific diseases.

The ancient herbal food supplements are completely different from modern drugs. They are compilations of intact plants or parts of plants, and comprise a profusion of components, a rich stew of molecules intended to enrich the human physiology in its entirety. There is no attempt to isolate individual molecules. Moreover, these formulations are not drugs, but rich herbal foods that are used as supplements to the everyday diet and said to produce overall health and well-being. Although there have been thousands of years of clinical observations – systematic use by doctors in their practices – there has not been (until recently) the type of lab work and systematic experimentation typical of modern medicine. Nevertheless, recent scientific experiments have shown these formulas to be effective, and to have virtually no side-effects.

Ayurvedic *vaidyas* assert that the effectiveness of these herbal formulations comes precisely from the richness of their mixtures. They are a deliberate attempt to maximize synergism: the components help each other move through the digestive system, arrive at the correct cells, penetrate the cell membranes, and achieve intracellular effects.

SCIENCE AND SYNERGISM

Recent research on vitamins and bioflavonoids has identified simple synergistic effects; for example, *combinations* of antioxidants may do more to stop oxidation damage and cancer cell growth than would the sum effect of the same substances acting alone. One reason suggested is that the sequence of natural complex plant products sets up a cascade effect, which counters the damaging cascades set up among free radicals (Fishman 1994). But such cascades may well represent just a narrow spectrum of the full range of synergies that plant compounds display. These have long been a consideration of *dravyaguna* which deals with much more complex synergisms.

Assertions about complex synergisms are essentially impossible to check through objective science. In fact the concept of the isolated active ingredient sprang up largely because modern scientific investigation works best in the simplest situations. It must use a fragmentary, reductionist approach. One aim of scientific investigation is to work on the simplest possible isolated systems.

This approach has a logical basis. With only one

---

*MAK-4's ingredients are: *Terminalia chebula, Emblica officinalis, Cinnamomum zeylanicum, Elettaria cardamomum, Cyperus rotundus, Curcuma longa, Piper longum, Santalum album* and *Glycyrrhiza glabra.* These are processed in an extract of *Eragrostis cynosuroides, Premna integrifolia, Desmodium gangeticum, Phaseolus trilobus, Teramnus labialis, Aegle marmelos, Oroxylum indicum, Ipomoea digitata,* and many other herbs.

MAK-5's main ingredients are: *Withania somnifera, Glycyrrhiza glabra, Ipomoea digitata, Asparagus adscendens, Emblica officinalis, Tinospora cordifolia, Asparagus racemosus, Vitex trifolia, Argyreia speciosa, Curculigo orchioides,* and *Capparis aphylla.*

type of molecule to work with, a scientist can clearly show cause-and-effect relations. If you put one type of molecule into your beaker filled with fluid and the fluid turns from colorless to green, you know what caused the change. If you put in two types of molecules and the fluid turns green, you cannot be sure if it was one molecule or the other, or a combination of both. The uncertainty increases exponentially as you add more ingredients. Thus, the objective, scientific approach to knowledge biases the investigators toward uncomplicated, isolated reductionist solutions.

Researchers long schooled in this reductionist approach feel uncomfortable when a complex formula such as MAK is shown to produce positive results, since they cannot identify the 'ingredient' that causes the effect. Their objective training makes it difficult for them to think holistically, even to consider that it might be all the ingredients at once, working together. They know they will never be able to unravel such complications in the lab. And the tendency is to think that if you cannot examine it through reductionist experiment, then it is not significant.

Yet there is no logical reason why substances composed of a single molecular type should be more effective than a carefully chosen combination of ingredients. There is nothing absurd about the idea that a combination of ingredients may produce synergistic effects that enhance effectiveness and reduce side-effects. In fact, this view seems to fit naturally with the inconceivably complex operation of the human body and the manner in which the body interacts with the natural environment. To use a musical analogy, the body is not a single instrument, hitting a single note. It is a symphony of thousands of different instruments (biochemicals) varying and combining in countless ways – all at once, all interactively. Just as individual notes produce a harmony with other notes, so every chemical reaction in a healthy body is functioning in harmony with every other reaction in the body.

It seems reasonable that, to move this entire symphony in a more harmonious direction, it would be most effective to intervene with complex and holistic substances – with supplements that could affect the whole symphony at once. For this, however, one needs some way of knowing what the formula should be in the first place, and reductionist scientific investigation cannot provide that answer. But even if research can-

not tease out complex synergistic mechanisms, it *can* assess overall results. The research evidence on Maharishi Amrit Kalash to date is wide-ranging, showing marked antioxidant effects and a broad spectrum of specific benefits for specific diseases.

FREE RADICAL SCAVENGING EFFECTS

Dr Yukie Niwa was one of the earliest free radical researchers, and has been active in the field since the early 1970s. At his Niwa Institute in Japan, he has tested over 500 compounds for free radical scavenging effects. Since Niwa is an immunologist, much of his research has focused on the excess inflammation often caused by the immune system.

To begin their examination of Maharishi Amrit Kalash, Niwa and his colleagues conducted a chemical analysis of herbs in MAK-4 and MAK-5. These analyses revealed a mixture rich in low-molecular-weight substances that are well-known antioxidants, including vitamin C, vitamin E, beta-carotene, polyphenols, bioflavonoids, and riboflavin (Sharma et al 1990, 1991b).

Niwa then conducted an experiment to measure MAK's antioxidant effect. His investigation involved the immune system's most rapidly reacting defense – the neutrophil. Once inflammation begins, immune system cells such as neutrophils overproduce free radicals and other ROS, causing extensive damage to healthy cells in the vicinity. Chemicals released by damaged cells encourage rapid transit by neutrophils and other immune cells to the inflammation site, quickly worsening the damage.

Niwa's study showed that, in the presence of MAK, this neutrophil 'chemotaxis' slowed down significantly. In addition, the multiplication of lymphocytes in their most aggressive form (blastogenesis) was also tempered. He also identified the specific reason why MAK-4 and MAK-5 had this tempering effect on the mechanism of inflammation. Both of them markedly scavenged the neutrophil leakage of the serious free radicals known as superoxide, hydrogen peroxide, and the hydroxy radical (Niwa 1991). According to Niwa, in fact, MAK scavenged free radicals more effectively than any substance he had tested previously.

Dr Jeremy Fields and his colleagues at the Loyola University Medical School in Chicago followed up on

Niwa's work. They focused on superoxide since it is the 'master radical' – the first produced and the precursor of both hydrogen peroxide and the hydroxy radical. Fields' group compared MAK with SOD, the enzyme designed specifically to scavenge superoxide. Human immune system cells (neutrophils) were stimulated to create superoxide, as if to kill an invader. MAK and SOD were used to scavenge the superoxide.

The results showed that both MAK and SOD, separately, were able to scavenge completely the superoxide molecules. This was not a surprising finding, after Niwa's work. The surprise was that MAK proved every bit as potent as SOD, milligram for milligram. Because MAK has so many components, Fields and his colleagues conducted tests to make sure that, in defusing the superoxide, MAK had not damaged the neutrophils themselves. Results showed the neutrophils still healthy and functioning normally (Fields et al 1991).

The implications were significant. First, the tests indicated that MAK can reduce the random damage caused by neutrophils as they fight invaders. Second, if MAK scavenged superoxide as effectively as the body's own enzyme (SOD), its anti-free-radical effectiveness clearly deserved serious attention.

Further experiments reaffirmed MAK's ability to scavenge superoxide (Tomlinson & Wallace 1991). Also, a separate study by Dr Chandradhar Dwivedi and co-workers at South Dakota State University showed that MAK-4 and MAK-5 were able to scavenge other dangerous molecules – lipid peroxides (Dwivedi et al 1991).

One of the authors (Sharma) and other researchers at Ohio State University College of Medicine designed and executed another systematic test of MAK, directly comparing MAK-4 and -5 with three individual antioxidants – vitamin C, vitamin E, and the well-researched drug probucol. We wanted to use quantitative measures to assess the dimensions of this apparent antioxidant breakthrough.

We ran our test on a third oxidant, low density lipoprotein (LDL) which had been oxidatively damaged by free radical attack. LDL is known as the 'bad' cholesterol, not owing to its natural state, which is benign, but to its transformed state after free radical attack. Oxidized LDL (LDL-ox) is capable of causing extensive damage, which is central to the process that

scars, thickens and stiffens arterial walls, narrowing the artery passageway and attracting platelets which can aggregate into clots and block the artery entirely. The research indicated that if LDL-ox could be scavenged effectively, cardiovascular disease could be markedly reduced.

For our experiments, we used LDL isolated from human blood samples, and added copper ions to begin a free radical chain reaction. Copper ions, like iron, catalyze a reaction that attacks the double bond in LDL and steals an electron, leaving the LDL altered and radicalized. Once the reaction has begun, it spreads from molecule to molecule of the LDL, in a self-perpetuating cascade, as each damaged molecule damages another.

One group of tests were run over two periods of time, 6 hours and 24 hours, after which the incubation mixtures were frozen to stop the reactions. In a different series of tests, the herbal food supplements, vitamins C and E, and probucol were added individually to test tubes containing LDL and copper ions. These substances were also added to test tubes containing LDL without the copper ions. The various substances were added to the test tubes at 0 hours, after 1.5 hours, and after 3.5 hours; the incubation of the tubes was continued for a total of 24 hours. As an experimental control, a parallel set of tubes was run which did not contain the antioxidant substances.

Since MAK-4 is a thick paste and MAK-5 a tablet, aqueous and alcoholic extracts were made by dissolving the two supplements in an aqueous and an alcoholic solution.

As expected, vitamins C and E, probucol, and MAK all prevented the radicalization of LDL if added at time zero. All stopped the ongoing free radical chain reactions if added after 1.5 or 3.5 hours. But the difference in potency was startling. Weight for weight, the aqueous extracts of MAK were several hundred times more potent than vitamins C and E and probucol, while the alcoholic extracts were even stronger – at least 1000 times more potent.

In the same study we also tested two other MAV herbal formulas. MA-631 is described as similar in purpose to the MAK formulas; Maharishi Coffee Substitute is a herbal beverage. Each scavenged LDL-ox radicals with a relative effectiveness that was close to that of MAK (Sharma et al 1992).

DOES MAK BENEFIT HEALTH?

The above research indicates that there is now an effective means to protect LDL against free radical attack. If this is true, it means there are natural food supplements that can help keep arteries clear and work adjunctively to prevent a high percentage of heart disease, stroke, and generalized oxygen starvation throughout the body.

These findings are consistent with a large body of research. As this text goes to press, nearly 40 studies have been done on MAK worldwide, research conducted by at least 50 investigators representing a broad range of universities and independent research institutions. These studies have painted a consistent picture.

If MAK is an effective free radical scavenger, it should enhance health in a significant way. Laboratory and animal studies and human trials have given evidence that MAK's antioxidant effects translate into specific benefits for specific disease. The details give a picture of the possibilities available from synergistic free radical management.

Enhancing immunity

A sound immune system is vital to continued health. For this reason, a number of studies have focused on immune function. Both MAK-4 and MAK-5 increase the responsiveness of lymphocytes and MAK-5 increases the responsiveness of macrophages. Both results can be understood in terms of reduced free radical damage.

Researchers at the University of Kansas Medical Center collaborated with others at the Indiana University School of Medicine and with one of us (Sharma) at Ohio State University to conduct a study on the immune system in laboratory animals. One group of animals received MAK-5 in their diet for 20 days, a second group, serving as controls, did not. Under laboratory conditions, animals fed MAK-5 produced 32–88% more lymphocytes than the control animals (Dileepan et al 1990). This capacity for increased lymphocyte generation persisted for 15 days after MAK was removed from the diet.

Two subsequent studies revealed further immunity-enhancing properties of MAK-5, as well as of MAK-4. A follow-up study by the researchers at the University of Kansas Medical Center showed that lymphocytes from mice fed MAK-5 proliferated significantly more than those from mice which were not fed MAK-5 (Dileepan et al 1993). A study by researchers at the Gifu University School of Medicine in Japan showed that both MAK-4 and MAK-5 yielded significantly greater proliferation of lymphocytes from mice fed either MAK-4 or MAK-5 (Inaba et al 1995). This indicates that MAK-4 and MAK-5 may increase the responsiveness of the immune system.

The University of Kansas follow-up study also showed that macrophages from mice fed MAK-5 showed a significantly greater ability to destroy tumor cells when stimulated by two separate biochemical activators. In addition, the production of nitric oxide was significantly higher in the activated macrophages from the mice fed MAK-5. Nitric oxide is considered an important mediator in the process used by macrophages to destroy bacteria and tumor cells.

The effect of MAK-5 on the immune system was also indicated in a study on humans by Dr Jay Glaser, Medical Director of the Maharishi Ayur-Veda Health Center in Lancaster, Massachusetts. Many common allergic reactions are caused by excessive immune system response. White blood cells react to, say, a particle of pollen as if it were a deadly invading bacteria. The damage sown by these reactions results in inflammation of the nasal passage (hay fever) or the lungs (asthma). To test the effectiveness of MAK-5 on this type of immune system overreaction, Glaser randomly assigned subjects to two groups. One received MAK-5 and the other a placebo pill. Over the next 4 weeks, a peak allergy season, the group receiving MAK-5 showed significantly fewer allergic symptoms (Glaser et al 1988).

Controlling free radical effects on the immune system

MAK's effectiveness against free radicals can reasonably explain both the increased responsiveness of the immune system and the increased control of its tendency to overreact. Immune system cells are uniquely subject to damage. When oxy radicals and ROS released by immune cells damage their own membranes, their functioning is compromised. Cell receptors are damaged (Bendich 1990), reducing the responsiveness of each cell and the immune system as a whole to the body's wide variety of floating chemical messengers (Erickson et al 1983). Loss of membrane fluidity and destruction of protein machinery embedded in the cell membrane also cause decreased ability of the immune cells to respond to a challenge (Fountain & Schultz 1982). Thus, if free radical damage can be significantly controlled, increased responsiveness by the immune system should come about as a natural result.

Free radicals may also cause the immune system to spiral out of control. In the inflammatory response, oxy radicals and ROS overreact, and the damage feeds on itself by attracting more and more hyperexcited inflammatory cells into the fray. Antioxidants can temper this tendency to self-inflicted damage by rapidly scavenging the excess free radicals released by the neutrophils and other cells. The neutrophils, macrophages, and other immune cells can ingest and destroy toxic invaders without causing as much damage to their surroundings – and without attracting an excessive number of their cohorts.

The initial laboratory tests on MAK indicate the presence of both effects. The immune system becomes more responsive and more controlled at the same time. This shows promise for the control of both external (infectious) and internal (degenerative and inflammatory) disease. With the rich variety of molecules in MAK, there may be other mechanisms also involved, including the mind-body effects mediated through the limbic system in the brain (Ch. 4) and other mechanisms discussed below. MAK's free radical mediating capabilities may be one explanation for these immune system findings.

Cancer prevention and regression

Cancer may be tied to free radical damage, and thus has been another major area of MAK research. MAK has been observed to have certain antineoplastic (anticancer) properties.

Prevention and regression of breast carcinoma

The first cancer studies were on breast carcinoma, carried out as a joint project in laboratories at Ohio State University College of Medicine and South Dakota State University.

Carcinogenesis is ordinarily thought of as a two-step process: (1) an apparently irreversible initiation stage, when alterations occur in the DNA of one or more cells; and (2) a promotion stage, in which the population of initiated cells expands. Free radicals are active in both of these phases (Fischer et al 1988, Floyd 1990).

The initiation phase is related to chronic inflammation, an observation that has been made for many years but has only recently been explained. In chronic inflammation, white blood cells are constantly releasing showers of free radicals. The neutrophils and macrophages release superoxide and hydrogen peroxide in all directions, and both can enter nearby cells and travel to the cell nucleus to damage genetic material. Hydroxy radicals and hypochlorous acid released in intercellular spaces have the same effect indirectly. They attack cell membranes externally, giving rise to a chain reaction of radicalized lipids and the eventual production of aldehydes that can travel inward to the nucleus, where they crosslink DNA and its surrounding proteins (Weitzman et al 1985, Southorn & Powis 1988).

As for the promotion phase, there is evidence that cancer cells generate free radicals and ROS which speed their metastasis, or breakthrough from a local area to distant sites. Cells isolated in the laboratory from various types of tumors have recently been shown to produce copious flows of hydrogen peroxide. There is also indirect evidence that cancerous cells still living in the body produce free radicals and ROS; and aggressive tumor cell populations show increased production of antioxidants, indicating a need to protect themselves against self-generated free radicals (Borunov et al 1989).

In the first cancer experiment, laboratory animals were fed a diet supplemented with 0.2% MAK-5. They were also exposed to a potent chemical inducer of breast cancer: 7, 12 dimethylbenz(a)anthracene (DMBA). An 'initiation phase' group of animals received MAK-5 for one week before and 1 week after DMBA was administered. A 'promotion' group received MAK-5 1 week after DMBA administration until the end of the experiment. A third combined group was given MAK-5 throughout the experiment. After 18 weeks, only 25% of the animals receiving MAK-5 during the promotion phase showed tumors, as compared to 67% of the animals in the control group. However, there did not appear to be comparable protection during the initiation phase (Sharma et al 1991a).

A second experiment with the same design used a diet supplemented with 6% MAK-4. The animals on MAK-4 suffered 60% fewer tumors in the initiation stage and 88% fewer tumors in the promotion phase as compared to controls. In addition, in both studies, control animals who had already developed fully formed tumors were given the MAK diet. In 60% of these animals in both studies, the tumors shrank significantly. In roughly half of those that experienced this tumor regression, the tumor disappeared completely. The animals experiencing tumor regression were those that initially had tumors under a certain size; animals with tumors over this size did not improve (Sharma et al 1990, 1991a).

Reduction of aggressive lung cancer metastases

Another study was carried out on lung cancer by Dr Vimal Patel at Indiana University in collaboration with one of us (Sharma) and others. Patel chose Lewis lung carcinoma, known to be a cancer which aggressively metastasizes, spreading rapidly to other organs of the body. Rapidly metastasizing cancer is ordinarily the most life-threatening type. This study began with animals that already had Lewis lung carcinoma. MAK-4 was added to their diet. In 65% of the animals the total number of metastatic nodules decreased, and in 45% the size of the individual nodules also decreased (Patel et al 1992).

Increased survival

Dr Brian Johnston and his colleagues at SRI International (formerly the Stanford Research Institute) studied the effect of MAK on skin tumors, measuring increased survival rather than measuring effects on specific tumors. Animals with skin papilloma were fed MAK-5 in their diet. The survival rate for MAK-fed animals was 75%, as compared to 31% in the control group (Johnston et al 1991).

Prevention of cell transformation

In research supported by the National Cancer Institute (NCI), Julia T. Arnold, with colleagues at NCI

(Maryland) and ManTech Environmental Technology, Inc. (North Carolina), studied the anticancer effects of MAK with two standardized and frequently used tests. With one test, MAK-4 inhibited tumor cell growth by 51%. With the other, MAK-4 inhibited transformation of normal cells to cancer cells by 27%, and MAK-5 inhibited it by 53%. This was the first study to show specifically that MAK could prevent healthy cells from being transformed into cancerous ones (Arnold et al 1991).

Transformation of cancer cells to normal cells

The most striking cancer study showed the reverse process: cancerous cells being transformed back into apparently healthy, normal cells – one of the rarest types of reports in the research literature on cancer. It is often said that the initiation stage – damaging alteration to the DNA – is irreversible. This study – by Dr Kedar Prasad, Director of the Center for Vitamin and Cancer Research at the Health Sciences Center, University of Colorado – challenges that supposition. Prasad experimented with tissue culture cells of neuroblastoma, an aggressive form of neurological cancer most often found in children and considered extremely difficult to treat. Conventional therapies are known to create severe side-effects.

Typical nerve cells are by far the largest cells in the body, with large central bodies and branching dendrites and axions (long, fingerlike projections) which can be several feet long. Malignant neuroblastoma cells usually lose much of this nerve cell-style differentiation. They shrink, become circular, and lose their long projections. Once they have reverted to this small, nonspecific (undifferentiated) form, they begin to multiply uncontrollably. Prasad found that MAK-5 reverses this process. Exposed to MAK-5, approximately 75% of the malignant cells appeared to differentiate again, developing the large cell body and dendrites, and to stop their rampant growth (Prasad et al 1992). Their biochemical functioning also appeared to return to normal; they produced enzymes that healthy cells usually produce. Only a few agents had previously been reported which cause cancer cells to revert to a normal-like state, and most of them are highly toxic. We will discuss the implications of this reversal below.

Further scientific studies on cancer are now under way, but the reports already available have indicated that taking MAK as a herbal supplement may help prevent, reverse, or control some cancer conditions.

Reduced chemical toxicity

In modern society, many chemicals have become major causes of illness and death. This is true both of medications and occupational exposure. Much of the damage caused by these chemicals is due to free radical mechanisms. Exploratory studies have shown that MAK may have a significant role to play in this sphere as well.

Detoxifying adriamycin

For many cancers, adriamycin is a particularly effective medication. Adriamycin works by creating free radicals which destroy the DNA of cancer cells. However, these free radicals damage healthy cells as well. The danger is especially great in the heart, where cells have high levels of oxygen owing to their incessant muscular activity.

In collaboration with Dr Dwivedi at South Dakota State University, one of us (Sharma) together with colleagues designed a dual experiment to investigate whether MAK could reduce adriamycin's toxic side-effects. First, in a laboratory test, we checked to see if MAK could inhibit adriamycin's production of free radicals. Liver microsomes were incubated with a biochemical system that stimulates free radicals. In some cases, adriamycin was added to the system. Alcoholic and aqueous extracts of MAK-4 and MAK-5 were then added as well.

The first results showed that even in an already efficient biochemical system for creating free radicals, adriamycin increased the production of free radicals by 50%. Second, MAK again proved highly efficient at reducing free radical levels. The alcoholic extract of MAK-5 and both the alcoholic and aqueous extracts of MAK-4 reduced lipid peroxidation in the microsomes to essentially zero, even in the face of the added free radical load created by adriamycin (Engineer et al 1992).

An additional test was conducted on animals that were given adriamycin. One group was fed a standard diet, while the other groups received either MAK-4 or MAK-5. At the end of 4 weeks, the mortality among the control group was 60%. The MAK-5 group had a mortality rate one-third lower and the MAK-4 group had a mortality rate two-thirds lower. The results of these two experiments indicate that MAK may provide substantial protection against the toxic side-effects of adriamycin (Engineer et al 1992).

Protection against cisplatin

Cisplatin is a potent chemotherapeutic agent and is used successfully for treating testicular, ovarian, and other cancers. But it is toxic to the kidneys. This may reflect decreases it causes in the activity of the antioxidants glutathione (GSH) and glutathione-S-transferase (GST). One of us (Sharma), in collaboration with colleagues at South Dakota State University, studied the cisplatin-induced changes in GSH and GST in rat liver and kidneys. Cisplatin treatment significantly decreased GSH and GST activity in both rat livers and kidneys. But for rats who had dietary MAK-4 (6%) supplementation in addition to the cisplatin treatment, the effects of cisplatin on liver and kidney GSH and GST activity were reversed. These results indicate that MAK-4 may protect against cisplatin-induced toxicity (Sharma et al 1994).

Preventing toxicity in chemotherapy

Chemotherapy often destroys cancer cells by producing free radicals, which are not discriminating in their effects; they can sometimes even cause new cancers. It is not surprising, therefore, that MAK has been shown to be effective in reducing the toxic side-effects associated with chemotherapy. A non-random, controlled, prospective study on 62 patients showed reduced hepatic toxicity, vomiting, diarrhea, and improved sleep, weight, and overall feeling of well-being. They also showed a significant reduction in lipid peroxides compared to the control group (Misra et al 1994).

Protection against toluene

The *Charaka Samhita* says of a *rasayana* related to MAK-4 that, when used, 'even poison is reduced to non-poison'. MAK has in fact been found effective in protecting against such toxicities. In addition to reducing the often serious side-effects of chemotherapy and of anticancer drugs, it has been found effective in dealing with an industrial toxin. Dr Stephen Bondy at the University of California, Irvine, has tested MAK against the toxic effects of toluene, a hazardous industrial solvent. More than 2 million American workers are exposed to the dangers of toluene every day – dangers that result from toluene's ability to rapidly create free radicals. First, Bondy's laboratory tests showed that MAK effectively scavenged free radicals created by toluene. Next, a study was done on laboratory animals, which were first given MAK-5 for 2 days, then exposed to toluene. Examinations revealed a significant reduction of free radical formation in the MAK-5 group as compared to the control group (Bondy et al 1994).

Two other MAV *rasayanas*, Student Rasayana (Sharma et al 1995) and MA-631 (Hanna et al 1994), have also been found to reduce significantly toluene-induced toxicity.

Reducing cardiovascular risk factors

If MAK controls free radicals, it may also produce notable effects on atherosclerotic cardiovascular disease. Atherosclerosis contributes to heart attacks, strokes, and to generalized oxygen and nutrient starvation in tissue and organs everywhere in the body.

As we saw earlier, Maharishi Amrit Kalash has one potent effect that should markedly inhibit the development of atherosclerosis. MAK strongly protects low-density lipoprotein (LDL) from free radical attack (Sharma et al 1992). This would have obvious significance for treating and preventing atherosclerosis. If there are high levels of LDL cholesterol, much of that usually becomes oxidized by free radicals. This yields high levels of *oxidized* LDL, which clogs the arteries. Lowering cholesterol generally results in lowering oxidized LDL and oxidized lipids in general.

However, drugs used to lower cholesterol tend to have serious side-effects. Among patients who take anticholesterol medication, overall mortality rates actually go up slightly; and long-term use of cholesterol-lowering drugs may increase the risk of cancer

(Newman & Hulley 1996). Cholesterol has important bodily functions, including the production of hormones, bile acids, and cell membranes; too-low levels of cholesterol have been linked with depression. Besides, even relatively low cholesterol levels can contribute to heart disease if there remains a large amount of oxidation.

Thus the latest treatment strategy has been to give anticholesterol drugs in tandem with free radical scavengers. In the latter respect, MAK has been found to be effective. A clinical study at Ohio State University gave MAK-4 to hyperlipidemic patients; they showed significantly increased resistance to oxidation of their LDL (Sundaram et al 1995).

A number of other studies have found MAK to be effective in reducing atherosclerosis. In a study on rabbits with a strong genetic tendency to hyperlipidemia, MAK-4 reduced the average atheroma (deposit of lipid-containing plaque) on the aortic arch by 53% compared to a control group (Lee 1995). The most interesting finding of this study was that this reduction of atheroma occurred *without* a significant reduction in serum cholesterol levels – indicating that what reduced the atheroma was MAK's antioxidant effects. In fact, the study also showed that MAK significantly increased the resistance of LDL to oxidation (Lee 1995).

Other studies have found MAK and other MAV *rasayanas* to help prevent lipid peroxidation of various lipids, especially LDL; these results have been found with MAK, MA-208, Maharishi Coffee Substitute, and MA-631 (Sharma et al 1992).

Reduced platelet aggregation

Two more studies conducted at Ohio State have shown that MAK can inhibit atherosclerotic heart and vascular disease in another important way – by inhibiting blood clots due to the aggregation of platelets in the bloodstream.

Platelets normally promote blood clotting at the site of serious injury. But an excessive tendency to aggregate into clots can mean that platelets pile up inside blood vessels at sites of minor cell membrane damage and deposits of fatty streaks. This tendency toward excessive aggregation appears to be induced by four factors in the body:

1. Catecholamines, such as epinephrine and norepinephrine, which are increased during stress.
2. Collagen, which is exposed when cells lining the vascular walls are injured.
3. Arachidonic acid, which is released by membranes of injured cells.
4. ADP (adenosine diphosphate), which is released from injured red blood cells and platelets.

This chemical pattern means that if stressful living is combined with the type of damage free radicals typically do to blood vessels and bloodstream components, the conditions exist for development of clotting.

In one study, blood plasma from normal, healthy adults was obtained. Platelet-rich plasma was aliquotted into test tubes. All four inducers of platelet aggregation – epinephrine, collagen, arachidonic acid, and ADP – were tested. When an extract of MAK-5 was added to the plasma, there was marked inhibition of platelet aggregation (Sharma et al 1989).

Aspirin has become known for producing reduction in platelet aggregation and is now recommended for patients who have already suffered a heart attack. But aspirin has side-effects in the gastrointestinal tract and has been linked to an increase in brain hemorrhaging. Aspirin also has no effect on the aggregation caused by ADP. In fact, no previous study has identified a single substance which inhibits aggregation caused by all four of these inducers – and no significant side-effects from MAK have been reported (see below).

Reduced cardiovascular risk factors in living animals

It is one thing to get results in the laboratory. It is also important to see if the benefits carry over into living animals. In a study of two groups of animals fed a high-cholesterol diet, the basic cholesterol levels of animals given MAK were one-third less than those of the controls. In the MAK group, moreover, lipid peroxide levels in the blood (a measure of free radical damage) were nearly two-thirds less than controls. Finally, in blood from the MAK animals, platelet aggregation induced by collagen was 46% less, and aggregation induced by ADP 82% less. As reported in the experiment, MAK had substantially reduced these risk factors for cardiovascular disease (Panganamala & Sharma 1991).

Reduced cardiovascular disease

Does all of this translate into better cardiovascular health for human beings? Research suggests that it might. In 30 angina patients using MAK, there was a significant decrease in the mean angina frequency per month from nine to three attacks (Dogra et al 1994). In addition, systolic blood pressure fell, and exercise tolerance improved. The patients also reported improved sense of well-being while on MAK.

Anti-aging effects

One of the questions in free radical research is whether effective free radical control can slow the aging process and extend life. Three preliminary studies on MAK throw light on this.

Dr Jeremy Fields' team at Loyola conducted two of these experiments. In the first test, MAK was fed as a dietary supplement to laboratory mice, starting at the age of 18 months (roughly 50–60 years of age in human terms). Even starting at this relatively advanced age, 80% of the MAK group survived to 23 months of age, compared to only 48% survival for the control group. To check for effects throughout a life span, Fields turned to an experimental standby, the fruit fly. Fruit flies thrive and breed well in the laboratory, but their natural life span is only weeks long, allowing complete experiments in a short period of time. In this case, fruit flies fed MAK from birth lived 70% longer than controls (Fields et al 1991).

A provocative human test has also been conducted by Dr Paul Gelderloos and his associates at Maharishi University of Management in Fairfield, Iowa. Gelderloos reasoned that if MAK has a positive effect on aging, it should appear in measurements of age-related functioning. He chose a test combining both visual and mental processing in order to assess complex functioning of the nervous system. The test involves cards which have an array of letters laid out regularly in a grid. The grid contains 110 Xs and one V. The lone V tends to get lost in the sea of Xs. The Xs act as distractions (known as noise), attracting attention away from the target stimulus. Previous research on such tests had shown that the ability to quickly pick out the V worsens markedly with age (Gilmore et al 1985), owing partly to physical deterioration (such as reduced retinal metabolism) and partly to an age-related deficit in information processing (Plude & Hoyer 1985).

Gelderloos used a stringent research design. He first pair-matched 48 men for similar age and education, then randomly assigned one from each pair to one of two groups. One of the groups was given MAK-5, the second a placebo tablet manufactured to mimic closely the MAK tablet. Before the men started taking the tablets, they were given the visual test, with many variations of the Xs and V, each variation flashed on the screen for about three-tenths of a second. They were asked to locate the V and mark its location on sheets they were provided with. They were tested again after taking the tablets twice a day for 3 weeks, and again after 6 weeks. The experimenters and the people who scored the tests were not told which men were taking MAK and which the placebo.

The results supported the hypothesis. First, performance on the test, both for the MAK and placebo group, was strongly correlated with age. The younger men consistently scored the highest. Second, the group which took MAK improved significantly more than the placebo group in all age ranges after both 3 and 6 weeks (Gelderloos et al 1990).

Such statistically significant improvement in a matter of weeks would be difficult to explain were it not for the free radical theory. Long-range testing is still needed, but Gelderloos's work has demonstrated that MAK's free-radical scavenging ability may apparently rejuvenate cell function, thus improving a complex physical/mental process.

Redifferentiation and rejuvenation

In Chapter 3 the discussion of Transcendental Meditation touched on the dysdifferentiation theory of Dr Richard Cutler of the National Institute on Aging – the idea that cells 'forget' what specific type they are supposed to be. All cells in a body share the same DNA, but normally different genes express themselves in different cells. In aging and cancer, the cells regress (dysdifferentiate) to a generic and generally useless form. Cutler speculates that free radical damage to the DNA causes the dysdifferentiation.

This theory has relevance to the MAK research. Cutler has expressed the possibility that antioxidants might slow the rate of dysdifferentiation. The study by

Dr Prasad on neuroblastoma cells (mentioned above) has shown that, in certain circumstances at least, loss of differentiation may actually be reversed.

In Prasad's study, cancer cells incubated with MAK regained some apparently normal attributes of functioning. His study showed that as long as the newly redifferentiated cells continued to be cultured with MAK, they maintained their healthy, normal status. MAK appeared to help maintain their differentiation. This implies at least the possibility that regular use of MAK could help to maintain proper differentiation of bodily cells. If such differentiation continued in the most important glands of the body, which are Cutler's focus, then proper hormone levels would be maintained in the physiology as a whole. The aging process could be significantly retarded.

Mind and body

Intelligence

Research using laboratory animals suggests that *rasayanas* may influence mental function, partly because of their effectiveness in scavenging free radicals, but also because they increase a metabolite of arachidonic acid that enhances long-term potentiation, a process associated with learning (Sharma et al 1995). Dr Sanford Nidich and his colleagues at Maharishi University of Management found that the MAV herbal mixture known as Student Rasayana, in a randomized, double-blind study, improved the performance of children on a test of non-verbal intelligence (Nidich et al 1993). The experimental group showed an increase of nearly 10 IQ points on re-examination.

Emotion

In Chapter 4, we discussed the link between emotions and the body in terms of the limbic system and the neuropeptides it produces. Through this neurochemical system, emotions have a profound influence on the functioning of the body. We speculated that this is part of the reason for the physical benefits of Transcendental Meditation. Here we would point out that there is both logic and evidence for thinking that neuropeptides are modulated by MAK. For one thing, the Vedic tradition has always maintained that *rasayanas* enhance psychological well being. For another, if molecules are what mediate the mind/body interface, these particular molecules might be expected to mediate in a positive way.

To test the effects of MAK on both psychological mood and biochemical operations in the brain, we began with a much-utilized questionnaire that gauges emotional well-being. When given to people using MAK, the results of this questionnaire showed marked improvements in psychological mood – greater happiness, tranquillity, mental clarity, and emotional balance.

Was there any physiological explanation for these changes? To check for a molecular connection, one of us (Sharma) and colleagues investigated the interaction of MAK with receptors in the brain known as opioid receptors. Opiate drugs, such as morphine, attach to these receptors. There was much publicity a few years ago when researchers discovered that the body has natural opioids – endorphins and enkephalins – that also lock into these receptors. These can act as natural painkillers, and they also produce positive emotions, create a more relaxed and stable style of operation in the autonomic nervous system, and modify the functioning of the immune system.

These tests showed that MAK did in fact interact with these receptors: one or more of its components blocked the receptors for exogenous opioid compounds. However, it did not block receptors for *endogenously* produced opioid peptides. This suggests that MAK might be investigated for the treatment of substance abuse (Sharma et al 1991b).

Depression

A study carried out at Maharishi University of Management further implicated MAK's mind-body role. Imipramine is one of the major prescription drugs given for depression. It binds strongly with a receptor in the brain cells that increases the output of serotonin, one of the most thoroughly studied neurotransmitters. Low levels of serotonin correlate with aggression, hostility, and other mental health problems, while high levels correlate with a comfortable, even exhilarated emotional tone. Imipramine, the serotonin trigger, binds not only to brain cells but also to blood platelets, providing another tie between mind and body.

This research showed that MAK interacted with the same receptor on blood platelets as imipramine. This suggests that MAK might bind to the same receptor in brain cells, increasing serotonin levels and thus providing a positive effect on both psychological mood and immune system functioning (Hauser et al 1988). Further research is indicated.

Reducing inflammation and pain

A separate study reported that subjects using MAK-5 for 3 months showed a significant decrease in substance P, another neurotransmitter. Substance P is triggered by pain and is associated with pulmonary and gastrointestinal inflammation. Reduction of substance P thus indicates that MAK may be able to reduce such inflammation and its associated pain (Sharma et al 1991b).

These studies go beyond the free radical theory and indicate that MAK may have effects on consciousness as well as on the physiology.

Side-effects

Our experience with modern medicine has taught us always to look for negative results along with the positive. While modern drugs have side-effects, plants produce not only defenses against pathogens, but also toxins to deter predators; they can be toxic to people as well. Ayurveda has long asserted that *rasayanas* have no side-effects, that its time-tested herbal pharmacology has already dealt with the issue of toxicity and eliminated it. Beyond that, the mixture of components in *rasayanas* is said to increase potency, while also balancing biochemical influences and thus negating destructive side-effects. (This balancing effect of multiple ingredients is exactly what is lost with the active ingredient approach; active ingredients act indiscriminately throughout the body.)

To measure toxicity, a blood examination was carried out on 84 subjects who had been using MAK for at least 6 months. Standard tests of biochemical, hematological, and liver enzyme parameters revealed no toxic effects (Blasdell et al 1991). A separate study performed the same blood tests on nine subjects tested before and after taking MAK-5 for 3 months. Again the blood samples were normal and no toxic effects were found (Sharma et al 1991b).

Summary

MAK challenges some preconceptions of modern bio-medical science. It is a non-reductive mélange of thousands of different molecules, but it has passed some important scientific tests and produced measurable results.

It has been shown that MAK can help control free radicals, thus reducing the constant load of oxidative stress in the body and improving physical health in many measurable ways. The studies indicate that it works more effectively than many of the best-known antioxidants, and that it may help to combat a wide range of diseases.

MAK includes natural antioxidants – vitamins, beta-carotene, polyphenols, and bioflavonoids – in high concentration. It also includes a myriad of substances not yet isolated and examined in the laboratory. While modern medicine leans toward isolated active ingredients, usually produced artificially, Ayurvedic *vaidyas* maintain that complex herbal mixtures of properly chosen and prepared ingredients are more effective. They maintain that the natural synergism not only increases the mixture's potency, but also works to mitigate side-effects caused by individual components.

In the case of free radicals, and the wide-ranging damage free radicals may cause, the research on MAK apparently upholds the Ayurvedic view. To the extent that these studies are accurate, therefore, they help define a significant new modality for prevention and treatment of disease. They also may amount to a breakthrough in medical theory. Confronted with a basic common cause of illness and aging, free radicals, scientists have shown that isolated active ingredients – magic bullets – may not work as well as rich natural formulations. An emerging, deeper understanding of the causes of disease is beginning to lead to demonstration of the benefits produced by natural synergism.

USES OF OTHER HERBS

Single herbs

We have spent a great deal of time on the issue of *rasayanas*, partly because the research is significant, and partly because it throws the issue of active ingredients into particularly sharp focus. We do not intend however, to give the impression that *rasayanas* like

MAK are the only use of herbs found in Ayurveda, which has an extensive herbal pharmacopeia.

MAV uses herbs in a number of formulations based upon ancient Ayurveda. Some are taken everyday, the herbs being added to the patient's diet. As we saw in the chapter on diet, the different taste groups are said to affect the balance of the *doshas* in different ways; herbs and spices are often, by this scheme, used to balance the *doshas* and the effects of diet. In addition, many individual herbs are held to have specific medical effects. These are understood in a systematic way, using the categories discussed in the diet chapter: the system involves not only taste group, but also 'potency' (*virya*) – that is, whether the herb is heating or cooling – and specific qualities (*gunas*).

As an example of how this might be used, we will consider the Ayurvedic herb *ashwagandha (Withania somnifera)*. A MAV *vaidya* would note that this herb has three tastes, bitter, astringent, and sweet; its potency (*virya*) is hot; its aftertaste (*vipaka*) is sweet. He or she would also note the specific qualities associated with *ashwagandha*: it is said to alleviate *Vata* and *Kapha*; to be a diuretic and sedative; to increase sperm count; and to be useful against edema, cough, skin disease, leucoderma and other disease. It is also regarded as a general tonic (a *rasayana*).

Such analyses are also applied to more common herbs. Fresh ginger root, for example, has a pungent taste, but a sweet aftertaste; its *virya* is hot; it alleviates *Vata* and *Kapha*, but increases *Pitta* mildly. It is widely used in MAV remedies. For instance, it is used to enhance digestive strength (to strengthen the digestive fire or *jatharagni*), which, as we have seen, is a central element of health in MAV. It is also said to be helpful in fighting colds, anorexia (because it can be used in specific preparations to stimulate appetite and digestion), chronic arthritis, and constipation (for this, the ginger is dried and powdered). Many other herbs, some of them not well-known in the West, others common, are used in various similar ways in MAV.

Herbs for treating specific conditions

Another major use of herbs in MAV is to treat specific imbalances and health problems. There has been a surprisingly large amount of research on this topic, with most of it being in Indian medical journals. To take one study at random, P. Khosla, D. D. Gupta, and R. K. Nagpal (1995) investigated the Ayurvedic claim that fenugreek (*Trigonella foenum-graecum*) is an antidiabetic. In a controlled study, they found that fenugreek produced a significant decline in blood glucose in both normal rats and rats with alloxan-induced diabetes. Another study appeared in the *Lancet* in October, 1988, and included among its authors Baruch S. Blumberg, who won the 1976 Nobel Prize in Medicine for discovering the marker for the hepatitis B virus (Thyagarajan et al 1988). This study tested the *Phyllanthus amarus*, which 'was described in Indian Ayurvedic literature more than 2000 years ago' as being useful for the treatment of jaundice and other diseases. The plant was given for 30 days to patients with hepatitis B; within 15 to 20 days of the end of treatment, 59% of the treated patients had lost hepatitis B surface antigen compared with 4% of controls. The study also demonstrated a lack of toxic side-effects from the plant.

In spite of such studies, there has been little research and marketing of natural herbs in the West. This is partly because of the active ingredient model discussed above, but also because such herbs are not patentable. Billions of dollars are invested by pharmaceutical companies in research into synthesizing the active ingredient and then testing it in the laboratory and clinic; but there could be no return on investment for similar research on natural substances. You cannot patent a plant. However, emerging research on herbal formulations is changing that orientation.

How else (besides antioxidation) might herbs work?

The antioxidant research explains a great deal of the effect of *rasayanas*, and also, as we saw, of Transcendental Meditation. It may explain part of the action of individual herbs used for specific illnesses or for general use. But clearly more is involved than free radicals. The neuroblastoma study we discussed above, for example, makes it clear that at least some of the anticancer effects of MAK are due to more than free radical scavenging. For a cancer cell to assume its former, healthy state, the DNA within the cell must have been reset. Free radicals damage DNA. Antioxidants by themselves simply stop the damage.

From the standpoint of MAV, this is not surprising.

Dravyaguna thinks of herbs as being like tuning forks, which 'vibrate' with and harmonize the functioning of different aspects of the physiology. This is based on MAV's understanding of the body as being not so much a hunk of matter as a dynamic and orderly pattern of knowledge, which is based ultimately on the underlying vibratory patterns of natural law in the DNA and, before that, in the quantum unified field. The vibratory patterns existing in plants are said to enliven those elements of the human physiology with similar patterns.

In the understanding of MAV, each molecule in a herb is actually an impulse of intelligence, a particular 'standing wave' in the underlying field of consciousness. When carefully chosen, these match the impulses of intelligence in different parts of the human body. When the mind and body go out of balance, there are disruptions in the natural sequence that leads from pure intelligence to DNA, RNA, proteins, and on to the complete physiology. One such sequence produces liver cells, for example, another the heart. Where a sequence is disrupted, disease can occur in that particular part of the body.

The herbal preparations of MAV are said to provide the correct impulse to 'reset' a particular sequence, to build a continuous bridge again from the unified field of pure intelligence all the way to the manifest, surface-level expressions of the body. When MAK encourages cancer cells to restore themselves to the healthy, functioning cells they once were, Ayurvedic *vaidyas* indicate that this process of redifferentiation means that the correct sequence is restored, the intelligence flows smoothly, and the *doshas* are rebalanced. We spoke in Chapter 2 about *pragya-aparadh*, the 'loss of memory' of the unified field; the research here suggests that cells too can 'regain memory' of their true natures.

SUMMARY

This chapter reviewed the body of research on MAV herbal formulas. This research gives reason to look beyond the 'active ingredient' model of modern pharmacology. A *rasayana* (a mélange of dozens of carefully chosen and prepared plants) was found to be 1000 times more effective at scavenging free radicals than the isolated active ingredients vitamins C and E and the modern pharmaceutical probucol. The mélange also proved to have a wide range of beneficial effects, many of which result from its antioxidant ability, but some from more profound capacities: restoring a cancer cell to normal functioning cannot be explained in terms of free radical scavenging. We speculated on the reasons for this in terms of the 'tuning fork' model used in MAV.

We also reviewed some of the wide range of other medicinal uses of herbs and plants in Ayurveda. This represents only a very small part of the herbal pharmacopeia. For this reason, we expect that the research covered in this chapter helps provide direction for more research (or more discoveries) to come.

REFERENCES

Alpha-Tocopherol, Beta Carotene Cancer Prevention Study Group 1994 The effect of vitamin E and beta carotene on the incidence of lung cancer and other cancers in male smokers. New England Journal of Medicine 330(15):1029–1035

Arnold J T, Wilkinson B P, Korytynski E A 1991 Chemopreventive activity of Maharishi Amrit Kalash and related agents in rat tracheal epithelial and human tumor cells. Proceedings of the American Association for Cancer Research 32:128 (abstract)

Bendich A, 1990 Antioxidant nutrients and immune functions. In: Bendich A, Phillips M, Tengerdy R P (eds) Antioxidant nutrients and immune functions. Plenum, New York, pp 1–12

Blasdell K S, Sharma H M, Tomlinson P F, Wallace R K 1991 Subjective survey, blood chemistry and complete blood profile of subjects taking Maharishi Amrit Kalash (MAK). Journal of the Federation of American Societies for Experimental Biology 5:A1317 (abstract)

Bondy S C, Hernandez T M, Mattia C 1994 Antioxidant properties of two Ayurvedic herbal preparations. Biochemical Archives 10:25–31

Borunov E V, Smirnova L P, Shchepetkin I A, Lankin V Z, Vasiliev N V 1989 High antioxidative enzyme activity in tumors is a factor making the immune system 'out of control'. Bulletin of Experimental Biology and Medicine 107(4):530–532

Burton G W, Ingold K U 1984 Beta-carotene: an unusual type of antioxidant. Science 224:569–573

Ciba Foundation Symposium 65 1979 Oxygen free radicals and tissue damage. Excerpta Medica, Amsterdam

Cross C E, Halliwell B, Borish E T et al 1987 Oxygen radicals and human disease. Annals of Internal Medicine 107:526–545

Del Maestro R F, Bjork J, Arfors K E 1982 'Free radicals and microvascular permeability' in: Autor A P (ed) Pathology of oxygen. Academic Press, New York, pp 157–173

Dileepan K N, Patel V, Sharma H M, Stechschulte D J 1990 Priming of splenic lymphocytes after ingestion of an Ayurvedic herbal food supplement: evidence for an immunomodulatory effect. Biochemical Archives 6:267–274

Dileepan K N, Varghese S T, Page J C, Stechschulte D J 1993 Enhanced lymphoproliferative response, macrophage mediated tumor cell killing and nitric oxide production after ingestion of an Ayurvedic drug. Biochemical Archives 9:365–374

Dogra J, Grover N, Kumar P, Aneja N 1994 Indigenous free radical scavenger MAK 4 and 5 in angina pectoris. Is it only a placebo? Journal of the Association of Physicians of India 42(6):466–467

Dwivedi C, Sharma H M, Dobrowski S, Engineer F N 1991 Inhibitory effects of Maharishi-4 and Maharishi-5 on microsomal lipid peroxidation. Pharmacology Biochemistry and Behavior 39:649–652

Engineer F N, Sharma H M, Dwivedi C 1992 Protective effects of M-4 and M-5 on adriamycin-induced microsomal lipid peroxidation and mortality. Biochemical Archives 8:267–272

Erickson K L, Adams D A, McNeill C J 1983 Dietary lipid modulation of immune responsiveness. Lipids 18(7):468–474

Fields J Z, Eftekhari E, Hagen J F, Wichlinski L J, Schneider R H 1991 Anti-aging and oxygen free radical (OFR) scavenging effects of an anti-carcinogenic natural product, Maharishi Amrit Kalash (MAK). Journal of the Federation of American Societies for Experimental Biology 5(6):A1735 (abstract)

Fischer S M, Floyd R A, Copeland E S 1988 Workshop report from the Division of Research Grants, National Institutes of Health: oxy radicals in carcinogenesis – a chemical pathology study section workshop. Cancer Research 48:3882–3887

Fishman R H B 1994 Antioxidants and phytotherapy. Lancet 344:1356

Fligiel S E G, Ward P A, Johnson K J, Till G O 1984 Evidence for role of hydroxyl radical in immune complex induced vasculitis. Federation Proceedings 43(4):954 (abstract)

Floyd R A 1990 Role of oxygen free radicals in carcinogenesis and brain ischemia. Journal of the Federation of American Societies for Experimental Biology 4:2587–2597

Fountain M W, Schultz R D 1982 Effects of enrichment of phosphatidylcholine liposomes with cholesterol or alpha-tocopherol on the response of lymphocytes to phytohemagglutinin. Molecular Immunology 19(1):59–64

Gelderloos P, Ahlstrom H H B, Orme-Johnson D W, Robinson D K, Wallace R K, Glaser J L 1990 Influence of a Maharishi Ayur-Vedic herbal preparation on age-related visual discrimination. International Journal of Psychosomatics 37:25–29

Gilmore G C, Tobias T R, Royer F L 1985 Aging and similarity grouping in visual search. Journal of Gerontology 40(5):586–592

Glaser J L, Robinson D K, Wallace R K 1988 Effect of Maharishi Amrit Kalash on allergies, described in Maharishi Ayurveda: an introduction to recent research. Modern Science and Vedic Science 2(1):89–108

Greenwald R A, Moy W W 1979 Inhibition of collagen gelation by action of the superoxide radical. Arthritis and Rheumatism 22(3):251–259

Greenwald R A, Moy W W 1980 Effect of oxygen-derived free radicals on hyaluronic acid. Arthritis and Rheumatism 23(4):455–463

Halliwell B 1981 The biological effects of the superoxide radical and its products. Clinical Respiratory Physiology 17(Suppl):21–29

Halliwell B 1989 'Free radicals, oxygen toxicity and aging.' In: Sohal R S (ed) Age pigments. Elsevier, Amsterdam, pp 1–62

Hanna A N, Sharma H M, Kauffman E M, Newman H A I 1994 In vitro and in vivo inhibition of microsomal lipid peroxidation by MA-631. Pharmacology Biochemistry and Behavior 48(2):505–510

Hauser T, Walton K G, Glaser J, Wallace R K 1988 Naturally occurring ligand inhibits binding of [3H]-imipramine to high affinity receptors. Paper presented at the 18th Annual Meeting of the Society for Neuroscience, 14 November, p 244 (abstract)

Hennekens C H, Buring J E, Manson J E et al 1996 Lack of effect of long-term supplementation with beta-carotene on the incidence of malignant neoplasms and cardiovascular disease. New England Journal of Medicine 334(18):1145–1149

Hooper C 1989 Free radicals: research on biochemical bad boys comes of age. Journal of National Institutes of Health Research 1:101–106

Inaba R, Sugiura H, Iwata H 1995 Immunomodulatory effects of

Maharishi Amrit Kalash 4 and 5 in mice. Japanese Journal of Hygiene 50:901–905

Johnston B H, Mirsalis J, Hamilton C 1991 Chemotherapeutic effects of an Ayurvedic herbal supplement on mouse papilloma. The Pharmacologist 3:39 (abstract)

Khosla P, Gupta D, Nagpal R K 1995 'Effect of Trigonella foenumgraecum (fenugreek) on blood glucose in normal and diabetic rats.' Indian Journal of Physiology and Pharmacology 39(2):173–174

Kushi L H, Folsom A R, Prineas R J, Mink P J, Wu Y, Bostick R M 1996 Dietary antioxidant vitamins and death from coronary heart disease in postmenopausal women. New England Journal of Medicine 334(18):1145–1149

Lee J Y 1995 The antioxidant and antiatherogenic effects of MAK-4 in WHHL rabbits. PhD dissertation, Ohio State University, Columbus, Ohio

Misra N C, Sharma H M, Chaturvedi A et al 1994 Antioxidant adjuvant therapy using a natural herbal mixture (MAK) during intensive chemotherapy: reduction in toxicity. A prospective study of 62 patients. In: Rao R S, Deo M G, Sanghvi L D (eds) Proceedings of the XVI International Cancer Congress. Monduzzi, Bologna, pp. 3099–3102

Newman T B, Hulley S B 1996 Carcinogenicity of lipid-lowering drugs. Journal of the American Medical Association 275(1):55–60

Nidich S I, Morehead P, Nidich R J, Sands D, Sharma H 1993 The effect of the Maharishi Student Rasayana food supplement on non-verbal intelligence. Personality and Individual Differences 15:599–602

Niwa Y 1991 Effect of Maharishi 4 and Maharishi 5 on inflammatory mediators – with special reference to their free radical scavenging effect. Indian Journal of Clinical Practice 1(8):23–27

Niwa Y, Hanssen M 1989 Protection for life. Thorsons, Wellingborough

Omenn G S, Goodman G E, Thornquist M A et al 1996 Effects of a combination of beta carotene and vitamin A on lung cancer and cardiovascular disease. New England Journal of Medicine 334(18):1150–1155

Panganamala R V, Sharma H M 1991 Anti-oxidant and antiplatelet properties of Maharishi Amrit Kalash (M-4) in hypercholesterolemic rabbits. Paper presented at the Ninth International Symposium on Atherosclerosis, Rosemont, Illinois. USA, 6–11 October, p 188 (abstract)

Patel V K, Wang J, Shen R N, Sharma H M, Brahmi Z 1992 Reduction of metastases of Lewis Lung Carcinoma by an Ayurvedic food supplement in mice. Nutrition Research 12:51–61

Plude D J, Hoyer W J 1985 'Attention and performance: identifying and localizing age deficits.' In: Charness N (ed) Aging and performance. Wiley, London, pp 47–99

Prasad K N, Edwards-Prasad J, Kentroti S, Brodie C, Vernadakis A 1992 Ayurvedic (science of life) agents induce differentiation in murine neuroblastoma cells in culture. Neuropharmacology 31:599–607

Sato Y, Hotta N, Sakamoto N, Matsuoka S, Ohishi N, Yagi K 1979 Lipid peroxide level in plasma of diabetic patients. Biochemical Medicine 21:104–107

Sharma H M, Dwivedi C, Satter B C et al 1990 Antineoplastic properties of Maharishi-4 against DMBA-induced mammary tumors in rats. Pharmacology Biochemistry and Behavior 35:767–773

Sharma H M, Dwivedi C, Satter B C, Abou-Issa H 1991a Antineoplastic properties of Maharishi Amrit Kalash, an Ayurvedic food supplement, against 7, 12-dimethylbenz(a)anthracene-induced mammary tumors in rats. Journal of Research and Education in Indian Medicine 10(3):1–8

Sharma H M, Feng Y, Panganamala R V 1989 Maharishi Amrit Kalash (MAK) prevents human platelet aggregation. Clinica Terapia Cardiovascolare 8:227–230

Sharma H, Guenther J, Abu-Ghazaleh A, Dwivedi C 1994 Effects of Ayurvedic food supplement M-4 on cisplatin-induced changes in glutathione and glutathione-S transferase activity. In: Rao R S, Deo M G, Sanghvi L D (eds) Proceedings of the Sixteenth International Cancer Congress 1994. Monduzzi, Bologna, pp 589–592

Sharma H M, Hanna A N, Kauffman E M, Newman H A I 1992 Inhibition of human low-density lipoprotein oxidation in vitro by Maharishi Ayur-Veda herbal mixtures. Pharmacology Biochemistry and Behavior 43:1175–1182

Sharma H M, Hanna A N, Kauffman E M, Newman H A I 1995 Effect of herbal mixture Student Rasayana on lipoxygenase activity and lipid peroxidation. Free Radical Biology and Medicine 18:687–697

Sharma H M, Hanissian S, Rattan A K, Stern S L, Tejwani G A 1991b Effect of Maharishi Amrit Kalash on brain opioid receptors and neuropeptides. Journal of Research and Education in Indian Medicine 10(1):1–8

Southorn P A, Powis G 1988 Free radicals in medicine. II. Involvement in human disease. Mayo Clinic Proceedings 63:390–408

Stringer M D, Gorog P G, Freeman A, Kakkar V V 1989 Lipid peroxides and atherosclerosis. British Medical Journal 298:281–284

Sundaram V, Hanna A N, Lubow G, Falko J, Sharma H M 1995 Increased resistance of human LDL to oxidation in hyperlipidemic patients supplemented with oral herbal mixture MAK-4. Journal of the Federation of American Societies for Experimental Biology 9(3):A141 (abstract)

Thyagarajan S P, Subramanian S, Thirunalasundari T, Venkateswaran P S, Blumberg B S 1988 'Effect of Phyllanthus amarus on chronic carriers of hepatitis B virus.' Lancet 2, 764–766

Tomlinson P F Jr, Wallace R K 1991 Superoxide scavenging of two natural products, Maharishi-4 (M-4) and Maharishi 5 (M-5). Journal of the Federation of American Societies for Experimental Biology 5(5):A1284 (abstract)

Weitzman S A, Weitberg A B, Clark E P, Stossel T P 1985 Phagocytes as carcinogens: malignant transformation produced by human neutrophils. Science 227:1231–1233

Yagi K, Matsuoka S, Ohkawa H, Ohishi N, Takeuchi Y K, Sakai H 1977 Lipoperoxide level of the retina of chick embryo exposed to high concentration of oxygen. Clinica Chimica Acta 80:355–360

9

The rhythms of nature

DAILY ROUTINE

According to the 18th-century botanist Carl Linnaeus, a competent botanist should not need a clock; he or she should be able to tell the time just by seeing which flowers are opened or closed. Something similar could be said of a good astronomer. From a planet to an atom, nature is characterized by regular cycles. The sun will rise tomorrow at a time that could have been predicted thousands of years ago, and the robins will not suddenly decide to fly by night and sleep by day.

The time when your neighbors awaken, however, may not be predictable. Human beings are free to retire and arise when they like. This flexibility can blind us to the fact that our bodies, too, work best according to specific natural rhythms. A new branch of modern medicine, called chronobiology, is discovering that the human body is a finely tuned timepiece. It has 23- to 26-hour daily (circadian) cycles, lunar (15- or 30-day) cycles, solar (circannual – one-year) cycles, and cycles which follow the ebb and flow of the tides. These cycles influence almost every aspect of bodily functioning. A tooth is most likely to begin aching between 3 and 8 in the morning, and least likely to begin between 3 and 4 in the afternoon (Pöllmann & Harris 1978). A dose of corticosteroids will control a patient's asthma and improve the 'peak expiratory flow' significantly more if injected at 8 a.m. and 3 p.m., instead of 3 p.m. and 8 p.m. (Reinberg et al 1983). Diseases and their treatments affect us differently at different times of the day and of the year; a substance may be fatal at one hour and not cause serious harm at another.

Moreover, medical research is showing that keeping

unnatural routines can weaken the body's immune strength and general effectiveness. Some evidence suggests that night shift workers have more medical disorders, especially gastrointestinal complaints (Meers et al 1978, Akerstedt & Torsvall 1978); the latter study found improvements when the worker returned to day shifts. But since the invention of the electric light and the adoption of clock-regulated time, more and more of us maintain routines that break our bodies' innate synchrony with the rhythms of nature. Today, we can stay up late, work late, and deprive ourselves of sleep – with dire consequences for health and society (Leger 1994, Coren 1996, Webb & Agnew 1976).

One way in which Maharishi Ayur-Veda (MAV) promotes health is to bring one's routines into synchrony with nature's rhythms. Medicine is beginning to work out the clinical applications of chronobiology, but the Vedic approach to health has recognized this principle for millennia, and has determined in considerable detail how clinicians and patients can apply it. So thorough is MAV's interest in chronobiology that even its pharmacology concerns itself with choosing the optimum time of the day and year for picking specific herbs: plants, too, have biorhythms.

Below are some elements of how MAV attunes human biological rhythms to the rhythms of nature.

EARLY TO BED AND EARLY TO RISE

Henry David Thoreau once said: 'Measure your health by your sympathy with morning and spring.' MAV would add that through sympathy with morning one can *improve* health. Arising with the sun is a health measure. More specifically, MAV says that the hour and a half before sunrise is the most health-promoting time to arise, but, if this is too early, then it is best to come as close to it as possible. This only works, of course, if one retires early as well.

Western research might explain Benjamin Franklin's 'early to bed and early to rise' maxim in terms of biochemical rhythms. Consider the hormone cortisol, which regulates the body's metabolism and is the primary biochemical means of resisting stress (without it, almost any activity would overwhelm the physiology). As a result of the 24-hour cycle of day and night, the adrenal glands send forth different amounts of cor-

tisol at different times. The daily peak is in the morning in the last hour of sleep and first hours of waking; and while this rhythm is slightly influenced by exogenous influences, it is mostly endogenous (Minors & Waterhouse 1981, pp 141–148).

As with homeostasis, MAV relates the various biorhythms of the human body to underlying regulators of biological rhythm. These have their influence not only in the human body, but throughout nature in general, and involve the now-familiar three *doshas*. In the world around us, as well as in human life, the influence of the three *doshas* – *Vata*, *Pitta*, and *Kapha* – is said to revolve in a specific cycle. *Kapha* dominates first, then *Pitta*, then *Vata*. Examples of this sequence are found in annual human biorhythms and in the human life cycle in general. Our present consideration is how it works in the broader daily cycle. From about 6 (sunrise) to 10 a.m., the qualities we associate with *Kapha* dominate the environment; from 10 a.m. to 2 p.m., as the sun reaches its zenith and the day warms up, *Pitta* reigns; from 2 to 6 p.m., *Vata* dominates, and then the cycle begins again: as evening falls, *Kapha* dominates; in the middle of the night *Pitta* is more active for 4 hours starting at 10 p.m., and *Vata* from 2 until the next sunrise. From this standpoint, if one arises before sunrise, one is arising during a *Vata* period, and mind and body will reflect the best qualities of *Vata*, namely lightness, alertness, and quickness. The person will feel more alert and clear during the day. If, on the other hand, one sleeps long past sunrise, one is more likely to wake up with mind and body imbued with Kaphic qualities, such as heaviness, slowness, and dullness.

So much for the 'early to rise' component of Franklin's maxim. 'Early to bed' is important for two reasons. The first is obvious: in order to gain a sufficient amount of sleep, an early riser needs to retire early. In addition, sleep gained early in the evening is said in MAV to be more refreshing. This is because *Kapha* dominates the environment in the evening until about 10 p.m., and if one retires before this hour one's sleep will be easier to attain and more restful, because it will be dominated by *Kapha's* qualities of heaviness and tranquillity. After 10, *Pitta* dominates until 2 a.m., and then *Vata* takes over; in those periods, sleep may be harder to gain and less refreshing. This corresponds to a common experience of feeling drowsy in the early evening, at 8 or 9 p.m., and then getting a 'second wind' after 10 p.m.

Our hormonal cycles are bioengineered for early rising, and MAV argues that this relates to an overall pattern of nature; thus, it says, sleep gained after sunrise will not be as refreshing as sleep gained before midnight. Western medicine used to believe that 8 hours of sleep would do an equal amount of good whether taken by night or by day. Ayurveda has always held otherwise: day sleep, because it strongly increases *Kapha*, makes people feel duller or heavier, while night sleep is, in Charaka's words, 'the nurse of every living being'.

Patients used to retiring and rising late may imagine that a change in schedule is impossible. Our patients' experiences suggest otherwise. Readjusting a schedule is like moving from say, Montana to Massachusetts. In that move, there's a two-hour time zone shift, but soon enough you adjust to going to bed earlier. A 'move' of one's own schedule is easier to manage, in that the body is aided by its own hormonal rhythms. In fact, we have found that an early bedtime is helpful in treating insomniacs, the very people who one would expect to be least amenable to such a routine.

Early to bed and rise is one of the central MAV prescriptions for both prevention and treatment, and applies to almost any patient; its health benefits can be significant. There are, however, many other elements of the MAV advice on daily routine, involving such areas as eating and exercise.

DAILY ROUTINE AND DIGESTION

In addition to the issues raised in Chapter 7, MAV considers circadian and circannual rhythms to be important elements of healthy digestion and diet. The digestive fire, or *agni*, is held to be at its strongest at midday, when the sun is at its height and *Pitta dosha* is at its strongest. It is weak at night, and not yet at full strength in the morning. The purpose of eating, MAV holds, is to extract energy, order, and matter from food; one needs these most as one undertakes one's daily activities, but not when one sleeps. During sleep, it holds, is when the digestive system is more concerned with purification and detoxification, as is supported by research on the circadian activity cycles of the liver (Axelrod 1968, Radzialowski & Bousquet 1968) and kidney (Lambinet et al 1981).

Thus the main meal of the day should be at noon, when the sun is at its zenith; this is when the body is most able to digest a large meal. This does not mean that one should overeat; doing so can lead to drowsiness and poor assimilation. Breakfast should, for most people, be a relatively light meal, as should dinner. Eating a large dinner can contribute to a number of digestive problems, such as acid indigestion and aggravation of hiatal hernias; it also can detract from the restfulness of sleep.

This advice also applies to the types of food eaten. Dinner should, for most people, not include heavy, harder-to-digest foods. Chief among these are red meat, but other examples are curdled milk products, such as yogurt and cheese. A preferred dinner menu might include such easily digestible items as soup, cooked vegetables, and light grains.

MAV considers the ideal times of the three meals to be: breakfast, before 8 in the morning – that is, as early in the *Kapha* period as possible (earlier would be even better); lunch, as close to noon as possible (digestion is held to be strongest when the sun is at its peak); and dinner before 6 p.m. (that is, before the *Kapha* period begins). Obviously, these times are not always feasible, but the closer one can come to them, the better it is held to be.

MAV also has some advice regarding between-meal snacks. The digestive process itself is said to involve the sequence of *Kapha*, *Pitta*, and *Vata*. The first half hour or so of digestion involves the mouth and stomach moistening the food, which is *Kapha*-dominated; the next 90 minutes or so involve the digestive enzymes and acids and bile breaking down the food, which exemplifies *Pitta*; and the final stages involve the movement of the food through the intestines, which exemplifies *Vata*. It is considered important to let this sequence play itself out before beginning the digestive process again. If one's meal is in the *Pitta* phase of digestion, eating again – and initiating the *Kapha* phase as a result – will disrupt the process, making it less effective and taxing the digestive system. One should wait, therefore, 3 hours or so before eating again after a major meal. Sometimes the *Pitta* phase of digestion produces what is called 'false hunger', a feeling of hunger that is easily satisfied simply by drinking water; snacking at this time will disturb the digestive process.

All of the above must be balanced according to the patient's constitution, his level of physical activity and resulting caloric needs, and other factors. Seasonal factors also bear on diet; these are discussed in the second part of this chapter.

EXERCISE AND DAILY ROUTINE

Moderate exercise is considered an important part of the daily routine. 'Moderate' means to about one half of one's ultimate capacity. MAV considers morning the best time for physical exercise; the *Kapha* period from sunrise to 10 a.m. is ideal, in that exercise counteracts Kaphic tendencies. The *Pitta* period of day, around noon, is not recommended, in that it coincides with the main meal of the day; one should wait at least half an hour after exercise before eating, and at least an hour and a half after the meal before exercising. Also, exercise tends to heat one, and in hot weather midday is especially unsuitable for exercising. Afternoon is acceptable. The evening is not considered a good time for strenuous exercise, since it is too close to bedtime, although a walk after dinner is considered health-promoting.

Seasonal factors also bear on exercise, as discussed later in this chapter.

THE MORNING SEQUENCE: BEGINNING THE DAY WITH PURIFICATION

The general concept of the MAV morning routine is that the first morning activities should involve purification, removal of the waste products that have accumulated in the previous evening. 'Purification' may seem either a new or a quaint idea; it is in fact emerging as something of profound medical significance (see Chapter 10).

MAV recommends beginning the day by evacuating the bowels, a habit that one can culture. The idea is that one should begin the day by eliminating the toxins and waste products of the previous day. (The bowels are more likely to move at daybreak among those who eat their main meal at midday, in that the transit time from eating to elimination is about 18 hours.)

The routine then recommends brushing the teeth, gently scraping accumulated phlegm off the tongue with a special metal tongue scraper, and then gargling with sesame oil, followed by *abhyanga* – the warm sesame oil massage – and a warm shower or bath. All of these relate to the purification theme; *abhyanga* is said to gently remove impurities from the tissues, and a shower or bath, of course, cleanses in an obvious way. One should then meditate and eat a light breakfast.

Massage

A daily oil massage (*abhyanga*), according to MAV, has profound health benefits. Little research has so far been done on *abhyanga*, but Vedic tradition maintains that it promotes softness and luster of the skin, lubricates the muscles, tissues, and joints, and increases their flexibility. Moreover, by stimulating the tissues in the body, it is said to help keep impurities from accumulating in the system. The *Charaka Samhita*, the most authoritative ancient work on Ayurveda, further states that daily *abhyanga* makes one 'strong...and least affected by old age', and more able to handle strenuous work and accidental injuries.

Modern medicine is beginning to recognize that the skin is not just a barrier, but is also a major immunologic and hormonal organ. It is reasonable to speculate that *abhyanga* may influence the skin's contribution to immunity and hormonal balance. A number of studies have found significant benefits from massaging newborns, such as enhanced weight gain and responsiveness (Field et al 1986, 1987, Rice 1977). Again, aging seems to result in part from subtle losses of blood perfusion to key glands as a result of atherosclerosis in the vessels leading to those glands; perhaps daily massage in the MAV style increases perfusion.

In addition, preliminary research on sesame oil *abhyanga* is emerging. Dr Edwards Smith found that those who practice it daily have significantly less bacterial infection on their skin. This may have to do with the major component of sesame oil, linoleic acid, which makes up 40% of the oil. Linoleic acid is known to inhibit the growth of certain bacteria, especially pathogenic bacteria. Linoleic acid also is a powerful anti-inflammatory agent; some researchers have compared its potency to indomethacin. While no one has researched this implication, it may account for the experience of many patients who find that *abhyanga* helps with joint problems. Finally, linoleic acid appears to be an anticarcinogen; sesame oil has been shown to inhibit in vitro malignant melanoma growth (Smith & Salerno 1992) and human colon adenocarcinoma cell line growth (Salerno & Smith 1991).

Further, sesame oil contains antioxidants, and heating the oil – which is traditional in Ayurveda – has been shown to increase the antioxidants' potency (Fukuda et al 1986, Sugano et al 1990).

For those with *Vata* constitutional types, *abhyanga* is strongly recommended, because it offsets the drying effect of *Vata*; but everyone can benefit from this aspect of the MAV daily routine.

How to perform the daily oil massage

The daily oil massage (*abhyanga*) adds between 3 and 20 minutes to one's morning, depending on how much time one can spare, but it is well worth it. According to ancient Ayurvedic texts, *abhyanga* makes one stronger, better able to handle strenuous work, and less affected by the aging process. Patients who perform *abhyanga* daily report an increase in strength, energy, and 'glow', and a better resistance to illness. The method is as follows:

1. Sesame oil is best for most people, because it settles all three *doshas* and nourishes the body. However, for those with a *Pitta* constitution, or if the weather is very hot, coconut oil, which cools down *Pitta*, might give better results. If sesame does not agree with you (e.g. if it causes acne), you may use olive oil in the cooler months.

Sesame oil has a unique value even from the standpoint of modern science, since its chemical structure gives it a unique ability to penetrate most surfaces. This is an important element of the oil massage. The ancient Ayurvedic texts make it clear that much of the benefit derives from the oil being absorbed through the skin. (Research in the last 30 years has confirmed that the skin can indeed ingest oily substances.) Sesame oil also contains unusually large amounts of linoleic acid (compared to coconut, olive, and other vegetable oils, which have fairly small amounts of linoleic acid).

2. The oil should first be 'cured' to make it more absorbable. This is accomplished by heating it to 220°F (use a cooking thermometer). Since any oil is flammable, a few commonsense procedures should be followed to avoid fire: (a) always heat oil on a low heat; (b) *never* leave oil unattended, not even for a moment, while heating; (c) remove oil from the heat as soon as it reaches the proper temperature, and set it in a safe place to let it cool gradually; do not refrigerate it at any point.

One usually cures a full quart or liter of oil at a time - an amount that will cover about 2 weeks worth of *abhyangas*.

3. Begin each morning's massage by heating a quarter-cup of the cured oil to slightly warmer than body temperature (100°F, for example). This is typically done by placing the container the oil is kept in – a plastic squeeze bottle works well – in hot water for a short while.

4. Start by massaging the head. Place a small amount of oil on the scalp and massage the scalp vigorously, using the open palms of the hands and the flat surfaces of the fingers rather than the fingertips for the whole massage. The stroke should be circular, describing *small* circles. Spend more time on the head than on other parts of the body, because, as Ayurveda explains, the scalp has vital points (*marmas* – see Chapter 11) which connect to and influence the rest of the body.

5. Massage the face and outer part of the ears, using the fingers. Massaging the ears is also said to influence the whole body, so give them some extra time, too, but don't massage them vigorously. At this point, you may want to apply the remaining oil over the rest of the body: this will give the maximum time for the oil to penetrate the skin.

6. Massage the front and back of the neck, and the upper part of the back. Remember to use the open palm and flat surfaces of the fingers, not the fingertips, for most of the massage.

7. Next, massage the arms vigorously. For the joints use a circular motion, and for the long bones a straight motion.

8. Now do the chest and stomach. Be less vigorous here. Use a circular motion over the pectoral areas, and a straight motion over the breastbone. Then massage very gently over the solar plexus in a straight motion. Use a very gentle circular motion over the abdomen, moving clockwise, the direction the large intestine moves in.

9. Massage the back and spine – or what you can reach of it – vigorously.

10. Vigorously massage the legs in the same way you did the arms: straight on the bones, circular on the joints.

11. Last but not least, massage the feet. The soles of the feet are said to have *marma* points which connect to the rest of the body, so give extra time and attention to them. Once again use the palm or the open flat of the hand, and massage vigorously.

12. The ideal length of a daily *abhyanga* is 10 to 20 minutes, but it is better to give it only 2 or 3 minutes than to skip it entirely.

Be careful about getting oil over your bathroom floor. If your bathroom is carpeted, we suggest that you protect it with a tarpaulin, an inexpensive floor mat, or disposable plastic lawn or trash bags.

Oil gargle

After the oil massage is the best time to shave and to cut the nails if necessary. Then comes another step that is new to most of us: the oil gargle. This is said to help prevent dental problems (especially periodontal or gum disease) and also to protect the throat from soreness. Moreover, it is said to enliven the taste buds. Dr Mary Martha Stevens, Chairperson of the Dental Hygiene Department of Wichita State University, found that people who used this gargle daily had significantly lower ($p < 0.001$) bacteria colony types in subgingival probe specimens (Stevens 1989). If further research supports this finding, dentists may someday include this procedure among strategies for saving teeth from periodontal disease and decay.

How to perform the oil gargle

1. Rinse the mouth and throat with warm water. Take a mouthful of warm sesame oil; hold it for 2 minutes in the mouth.
2. Spit out the oil, then take a half mouthful of oil. Gargle for a minute or two, stopping for breath when necessary. Spit out.
3. Using a finger, massage the gums with sesame oil for a minute or so. One need only massage the part

of the gum that is in front of the teeth, not the part behind them.

4. Rinse the mouth and throat with warm water again.

Bath

The next step is to bathe or shower. In the heat of summer, one should use cooler water, but most of the year warm water is better. MAV recommends that one use a very mild vegetable oil-based soap (and shampoo), one that will not remove all the oil from the pores, so that the oil can continue to benefit the skin. The milder the soap, the better for general skin care. The ancient Ayurvedic practice was to use not soap but barley or chick pea flour, which soaks up the oil from the surface but leaves it in the pores. If you try these flours, however, be careful that they don't clog your drains.

Ayurveda does not recommend using hot water on the head, especially for those with a *Pitta* body type. For the head, use lukewarm or slightly warm water.

Meditation

The next step in the routine, after *abhyanga* and showering, is Transcendental Meditation (Ch. 3). The benefits of TM are cumulative, and are maximized by regular daily practice, in which the two daily meditation periods – morning and early evening – are followed by activity, which stabilizes the benefits of meditation, and which is itself enriched by meditation. Patients often find that practicing TM early in the evening refreshes them so significantly that they, as several have put it, 'get their evenings back' – they have more energy and alertness to enjoy evening activities with.

DAILY ROUTINE IS IN AND OF ITSELF BENEFICIAL

Patients may or may not want to adopt all of the above elements into their routine (to prioritize, Transcendental Meditation is by far the most important). Whatever they do adopt, one point to remember is that routine is in and of itself beneficial. The body is designed to operate according to 24-hour cycles; whatever one's routine, routinizing it is in itself health-promoting. But the above principles can make the routine significantly more healthful.

SEASONAL ROUTINE

We have seen how our biorhythms connect to the earth's most obvious rhythm, its daily rotation. They connect also to another rhythm – the earth's journey around the sun, the year. The year influences us most through the many factors, such as weather, length of day, and flora, that change with the seasons. Seasonal transitions challenge the body; they cause minor illnesses and contribute to larger ones. By adjusting the patient's routine to the season, MAV aims to keep the body in balance, and thus reduce colds, sore throats, and other seasonal ailments, while maximizing strength and vitality.

Modern science, which has been studying daily biological rhythms for years, is only beginning to consider annual rhythms. Researchers have found that the levels of certain key hormones vary with the seasons. Medicine also knows that some people become depressed in the winter, in what is called Seasonal Affective Disorder Syndrome. Ayurveda has discussed the seasons' effects for thousands of years. Its knowledge is detailed and of immediate clinical value.

THE THREE SEASONS

In North America and Europe we take four seasons for granted. But in parts of Asia people are used to six. In addition to our four, they have a rainy season at the end of summer and a dry (as well as a wet) winter. And there are other possibilities: areas near the tropics or poles may have only one or two seasons.

MAV avoids the confusion by noting that the changes in our environment over the year affect the three *doshas* in a specific sequence. The first *dosha* to be aggravated is *Kapha*, by the springtime's moisture and coolness; the second is *Pitta*, by the summer's heat; and the third is *Vata*, by the cold winds of late autumn and winter. For this reason, MAV adjusts routines for three seasons: *Kapha*, *Pitta*, and *Vata*.

This sequence is common to many time passages.

Not only whole li of *Kaph* adults to do with ho ac r olde , and are more taking measures to co ful to the elderly. On the oth Vata, including subtle, refined insight, evident in old age (Box 9.1).

This ubiquitous sequence (*Kapha-Pitta-Vata*) reflects MAV's central theme, that the human body and the body of nature reflect each other (a Vedic maxim has it that 'As it is in the macrocosm, so it is in the microcosm'). Nature and the body are part of a single continuum of intelligence. This theme is the essence of how MAV handles the change of the seasons. Balancing the three *doshas* is the key to adapting to the effects of the seasons, since each season exhibits the predominance of one *dosha*. For example, the heat of summer is obviously *Pitta*; as we pass through this time period, we tend to absorb *Pitta*, and therefore the summer routine is designed to reduce *Pitta*. By contrast, the cold of winter increases *Vata* and *Kapha*, which are cold by nature. Since *Vata* is quick-moving, it becomes aggravated immediately; therefore, winter

---

Box 9.1 The seasons, times of day, and life periods classified according to the *doshas*

Kapha season: Spring–early summer (approx. March–June)
Kapha time: Approx. 6 a.m. (sunrise) to 10 a.m. and 6 p.m. to 10 p.m.
Kapha period in life cycle: Childhood

Pitta season: Midsummer–early autumn (approx. July–October)
Pitta time: Approx. 10 a.m. to 2 p.m. and 10 p.m. to 2 a.m.
Pitta period in life cycle: Adulthood

Vata season: Late autumn–winter (approx. October–February)
Vata time: Approx. 2 a.m. to 6 a.m. (sunrise) and 2 p.m. to 6 p.m.
Vata period in life cycle: Old age

...reducing diet and routine.
...wly, so spring – when the by-
...*na* is further aggravated by the
... is the time to reduce *Kapha*.
...ed review of MAV's recommenda-
...son.

...ason: March through June

...health-disrupting influence is partly the back-
...winter's effects. *Kapha dosha*, which gives the
...y its substance, is cold by nature, so during the
...ld of winter *Kapha* accumulates. When the weather
warms in spring, the *Pitta* 'liquifies' the accumulated
Kapha, which is then eliminated from the body. If there
is excess *Kapha*, it produces its *mala* or waste product,
mucus. As a result, in the spring patients tend to be
more susceptible to colds, nasal allergies, coughs,
sinusitis, and other respiratory congestion syndromes
– all signs of *Kapha* aggravation.

For these reasons, the MAV routine for spring
involves steps to reduce (and not further increase)
Kapha. Chief among *Kapha*-controllers is the *Kapha*-
pacifying diet, covered in detail in Chapter 7. In brief,
it involves taking more foods of the bitter, spicy, and
astringent taste groups, all of which reduce the qualities of *Kapha*, and fewer foods of the sweet, cold, oily,
heavy, and salty groups, all of which increase them.

How closely one should attend to this diet depends
on *prakriti* and *vikriti*. For *Kapha* types, or those with
Kapha imbalances, it will be extremely important. For
Pittas, it is less necessary. And *Vatas* may need to continue some *Vata*-(rather than *Kapha*-) pacifying procedures. Most patients, though, will probably need to
lean in the direction of pacifying *Kapha*.

To continue the list of *Kapha*-pacifying procedures,
during spring one should drink warm liquids only,
never cold ones. One should cover one's head when
there is wind or rain. Sunshine, which is warm and
drying, helps reduce *Kapha* (which is cold and moist).
Regular exercise, which reduces *Kapha*, is more important in the spring than at any other time.

Among the strongest health measures when spring
comes is *panchakarma*, Ayurvedic rejuvenation therapy
(see Chapter 10). Ancient Ayurvedic texts regard this
means of removing backlogged imbalances and impurities as being especially valuable at this time of year.

Spring routine

1. Minimize cold, sweet, sour, salty, or oily foods,
   and avoid cold drinks; favor warm food and
   drinks, and favor spicy, astringent, and bitter
   tastes.
2. Minimize daytime sleep, which increases *Kapha*.
3. Exercise regularly.

Pitta season: July through October

The obvious hazard of summer is that the heat aggravates *Pitta dosha*; a natural routine involves measures
to pacify *Pitta*. A key element is the *Pitta*-reducing diet.
This involves avoiding hot, spicy, and salty foods, and
favoring sweet, cooling, liquid, unctuous foods and
drinks. Notice that we often tend naturally to prefer
such foods in summer – ice cream, watermelon, cool
drinks – but many patients tend to ignore the injunc-
tion against spicy and especially salty foods at this
time of year; observing this is often helpful, particularly to those with *Pitta* problems.

Once again, whether or not to adopt the *Pitta*-pacify-
ing diet depends on the patient's constitution and
imbalances. Remember that the differences among
MAV diets are matters of degree. In summer most
people should take less of those tastes (salty, sour, and
spicy) that increase *Pitta* and more of those tastes that
pacify it (sweet, bitter and astringent). Some, however,
will have other needs; for example, those with
significant *Kapha* imbalances will have to minimize the
sweet food, even in summer.

According to MAV, the *agni* or digestive fire is weaker in very hot summer weather than it is in the cold
months. In the winter the body has to provide its own
heat, so the digestive fire is at its strongest, but in very
hot weather vitality in general is reduced by the sheer
intensity of the heat. Thus, most people should eat less
in summer, as many people find they naturally tend to
do. (Studies of rats have shown that spontaneous
caloric intake peaks in winter and is at its minimum in
summer, and some studies of humans have found the
same, though others have found slight variations; see
Reinberg & Smolensky 1983, p 268.) Note that this
advice does not apply to growing children, who
should not be put on diets or discouraged from eating
a healthy diet.

Also, although in the summertime cold drinks may be acceptable for *Pitta* types (and cool drinks for others), finishing a meal with them can douse the digestive fire.

Patients should exercise less in the summer, because exercise heats the body. MAV usually recommends daily exercise for everyone (according to individual needs) unless ill, fasting, or taking *panchakarma*, but in summer patients should cut down on the amount and intensity of exercise, and avoid exercise in the midday sun or afternoon heat. Swimming is a good summer exercise, because the cooling water helps pacify *Pitta*.

Like modern medicine, MAV recommends that one avoid excess exposure to the sun. The risks of skin cancer and premature skin aging are thought to be greater among *Pitta* types or those with *Pitta* problems. According to MAV, 10 minutes per day of direct exposure to the sun – the amount one would automatically get in the course of a normal day – is enough. MAV also recommends sunglasses on bright summer days; the eyes are one of the five main seats of *Pitta dosha*, and the summer sun can aggravate *Pitta* through them (modern medicine has also found that the UV radiation can lead to cataracts). For similar reasons, MAV recommends wearing a hat (or using a parasol) on a hot summer day. If you can avoid it, do not stay out in the midday sun. However, walks in the moonlight or by a garden, forest, or pool are soothing in summer.

One should bathe in cooler water than usual, though not in cold water. In summer, *Pitta* types may benefit from using coconut oil, which is cooling, instead of sesame oil for their daily oil massage.

Many patients have reported that *nasya* (MAV nasal therapy) at the beginning of allergy season can help prevent late summer allergies, which involve *Pitta* as well as *Kapha* aggravation.

Summer routine

1. Favor cool, sweet, bitter, astringent, and oily foods; minimize hot, spicy, salty ones.
2. Appetite may be reduced; don't overtax it.
3. Reduce exercise and sunbathing.
4. Swimming is a good exercise in summer, as is walking in the moonlight, forests, mountains, or gardens.
5. Wear a hat and sunglasses outdoors.

Vata season: October through February

According to MAV, what we call autumn is not one season, but the junction of two: *Pitta* and *Vata* seasons. *Pitta dosha* accumulates over the summer, so *Pitta* needs attention until middle or late October even if the weather cools slightly. Then a change occurs: cooler winds blow in, and *Vata* begins to dominate the environment. *Any* transition can aggravate *Vata*, and this transition is to a *Vata* atmosphere, so it becomes doubly important to keep that *dosha* balanced.

Note, however, that the enlivenment of *Vata* can have good as well as disrupting effects. It can, for example, increase energy, vitality, and liveliness – all the best qualities of *Vata dosha*. And the digestive fire, which is as it were hemmed in by the cold air, burns at its brightest, so digestive power is at its maximum. One may very well feel one's appetite increase in winter.

The problems of winter occur if *Vata* becomes aggravated or overly aroused, which is especially likely in *Vata* types. This can produce oversensitivity to cold, respiratory infections, insomnia, dry skin, indecisiveness, hyperactivity, and worry.

Vata dosha is cold, dry, and quick-moving. To control it, then, MAV favors its opposites, such as warmth and oleation. Regarding warmth, one should favor warm, well-cooked foods. One should not take cold drinks; drink warm liquids instead. The *Vata*-pacifying diet, which is a central factor in controlling *Vata*, emphasizes warm, unctuous (oilier) foods, and sweet, sour, and salty tastes, and suggests minimizing cold, dry, raw, rough, pungent, or astringent foods. The warmth the body creates radiates away through the skin, so keeping well-wrapped is essential for the *Vata* season. One should keep the head and neck covered on windy, rainy, or cold days, and avoid drafts especially – they aggravate *Vata* as few factors can. Indoor rooms should be comfortably warm. Since the air is dry to begin with, and central heating dries it further, a humidifier is often recommended, especially for *Vata* types.

Regarding oleation, daily *abhyanga* (oil massage) is particularly important in autumn and winter. Massaging the skin with warm sesame oil pacifies all three *doshas*, but the soothing influence of warmth and touch on the skin's many nerve endings calms *Vata dosha* especially. This affects the whole system, because *Vata* leads the other *doshas*, and, when it becomes aggravated, the other two often follow suit. Daily *abhyanga* will benefit anyone, but for *Vata* types it is particularly important, especially in winter. Apart from the benefits discussed above, *abhyanga* will keep the skin from becoming dry and cracked, a frequent problem for *Vatas* in winter.

Winter routine

1. Favor warm, well-cooked unctuous, sweet, salty, or sour foods; reduce cold, dry, raw, rough foods.
2. Keep out of drafts; cover the head and neck when outside.
3. Use a humidifier.
4. Do *abhyanga* daily.

Transitions between the seasons

The time when one season changes into the next is the most likely time for illness to strike (because any change aggravates *Vata*, and *Vata* 'leads' the other two *doshas*). For that reason, the routine recommended for a new season should be eased into gradually over a period of 1 or 2 weeks just before the new season starts.

CONCLUSION

Much of the advice given above simply reminds us of what we naturally do when we are alert to our body's needs and inclinations. In summer, we naturally tend to bathe in cooler water and to eat sweet, cooling foods. In winter, we naturally seek warmth in food, clothing, and shelter.

All the same, these reminders can help. How often do we neglect to put on a hat and scarf and to button up our overcoat in winter? And sometimes we get confused. Perhaps we think that if exercise is good for us, then more of it must be better – which is not necessarily so, especially in the heat of summer, when too much exercise could harm one. MAV clarifies these matters.

Though some of MAV's recommendations may be novel, they often become habit quickly. Patient compliance is higher than most clinicians would expect, simply because there is an immediate reward: patients feel better. For example, patients often enjoy the results of rising earlier. They discover that the reading, working or relaxing they used to enjoy until midnight are more enjoyable and productive in the early morning. This is an incomparably better time for a walk, for one can see, hear, and even smell the whole of nature waking up: its rhythms synchronize with one's own.

REFERENCES

Akerstedt T, Torsvall L 1978 Experimental changes in shift schedules – their effect on well being. Ergonomics 21:849–856

Axelrod J 1968 Control of catecholamine metabolism. In: Gual C, Ebling, F J G (eds) Progress in endocrinology. Proceedings of the 3rd International Congress of Endocrinology, Mexico City. Excerpta Med International Congress Series No. 184. Amsterdam, pp 286–293

Coren S 1996 Daylight savings time and traffic accidents. New England Journal of Medicine 334(14):924

Field T, Schanberg S, Scafidi F et al 1986 Tactile/kinesthetic stimulation effects on preterm neonates. Pediatrics 77(5):654–658

Field T, Scafidi F, Schanberg S 1987 Massage of preterm newborns to improve growth and development. Pediatric Nursing 13:385–387

Fukuda Y, Nagata M, Osawa T, Namiki M 1986 Contribution of lignan analogues to antioxidative activity of refined unroasted sesame seed oil. Journal of the American Oil Chemists' Society 63(8):1027–1031

Lambinet I, Aymard N, Soulairac A, Reinberg A 1981 Chronoptimization of lithium administration in five manic depressive patients: reduction of nephrotoxicity. International Journal of Chronobiology 7:274

Leger D 1994 The cost of sleep-related accidents: a report for the National Commission on Sleep Disorders Research. Sleep 11:100–109

Meers A, Maasen A, Verhaegen P 1978 Subjective health after six months and after four years of shift work. Ergonomics 21:857–859

Minors D S, Waterhouse J M 1981 Circadian rhythms and the human. John Wright PSG, Bristol

Pöllmann L, Harris P H P 1978 Rhythmic changes in pain sensitivity in teeth. International Journal of Chronobiology 5:459–464

Radzialowski F M, Bousquet W F 1968 Daily rhythmic variation in hepatic drug metabolism in the rat and mouse. Journal of Pharmacol Exp Ther 163:229–238

Rausch P B 1981 Effects of tactile and kinesthetic stimulation on premature infants. Journal of Obstetrics, Gynecological Neonatal Nursing 8:265–273

Reinberg A, Gervais P, Chaussade M, Fraboulet G, Duburque B 1983 Circadian change in effectiveness of corticosteroids in eight patients with allergic asthma. Journal of Allergic and Clinical Immunology 71(4):425–433

Reinberg A, Smolensky M 1983 Biological rhythms and medicine. Springer-Verlag, New York, p 268

Rice R 1977 Neurophysiological development in premature infants following stimulation. Developmental Psychology 13:69–76

Salerno J W, Smith D E 1991 The use of sesame oil and other vegetable oils in the inhibition of human colon cancer growth in vitro. Anticancer Research 11:209–216

Smith D E, Salerno J W 1992 Selective growth inhibition of a human malignant melanoma cell line by sesame oil in vitro. Prostaglandins Leukotrienes and Essential Fatty Acids 46:145–150

Stevens M M 1989 The effects of a sesame oil mouthrinse on the number of oral bacteria colony types. Presented at the 11th International Symposium on Dental Hygiene, Ottawa, Canada, June 1989

Sugano M, Inoue T, Koba K et al 1990 Influence of sesame lignans on various lipid parameters in rats. Agricultural and Biological Chemistry 54(10):2669–2673

Webb W B, Agnew H W Jr 1976 Are we chronically sleep deprived? Bulletin of the Psychonomic Society 6:47–48

10

Purification therapies: Maharishi Panchakarma

A car engine develops serious problems if dirt and grime accumulate in the oil, the fuel line, the carburetor, and so on. Although we've emphasized the problems of thinking of the body as a machine, in this case the analogy helps one to grasp how the functioning of the body suffers as impurities and toxins accumulate in the cells. Such impurities can come from both inside and outside the body. From inside the body come internal metabolic and cellular waste products, such as the free-radical-damaged cells discussed in Chapter 8; from outside come external impurities and toxins, such as pollutants (Rogan & Gladen 1992, Rogan et al 1988, Bahn et al 1976, Kimbrough et al 1975, Kahn et al 1988; Safe 1982) and toxins that occur naturally in food (Ames et al 1990a, 1990b). In Maharishi Ayur-Veda (MAV) terms, all these impurities (collectively called *ama*) block the body's inner intelligence. If left to accumulate, such impurities can lead to degenerative disorders and life-threatening disease. While the body has various self-purifying mechanisms, these prove increasingly inadequate as one ages, especially given the high level of toxins and pollutants present in modern industrial society. Like a careful car owner, we need to find a way to change the oil and filters on a regular basis.

Although Western medicine has for the most part focused its attention on putting substances (e.g. pharmaceuticals) *into* the body rather than taking unhealthful substances out, recently it has made some attempts to develop means of removing accumulated toxins from cells. These attempts have included the use of chelating agents, nonabsorbable resins (Nigro et al 1973), indigestible dietary fiber (Kritchevsky 1985), dialysis, and sweating (Schnare et al 1982, 1984).

Unfortunately, each of these approaches has drawbacks: side-effects (such as leaching important nutrients), limited effects (they only deal with a small part of the spectrum of accumulated toxins), and difficulty of implementation.

The MAV therapy known as *panchakarma*, we think, overcomes these problems. *Panchakarma* is a group of traditional Ayurvedic therapies designed to purify the body of impurities, and thus avert or reverse the development of disease and aging. *Panchakarma's* treatments are designed to first loosen impurities from bodily tissues, then eliminate them from the body altogether. Each treatment is individualized, depending on the patient's doshic balance and imbalances. Patients have consistently reported greater energy, clarity of mind, and well-being, as well as relief from a range of health problems, from back pain to arthritis to acne. Research also demonstrates significant benefits.

Panchakarma can be taken for as few as 3 consecutive days, and as many as 30. It can be done in residence or on an outpatient basis. It is most effective if done regularly – ideally, at the beginning of each season, to eliminate impurities gathered over the previous season.

HOW *PANCHAKARMA* WORKS

The word *panchakarma* comes from classical Ayurvedic texts, and means literally 'five actions'. This refers to broad classes of therapy used to remove impurities from the body. The classical texts – by Charaka and Sushruta – have slightly different classification schemes.

Although MAV Health Centers follow the Ayurvedic texts in replicating the traditional *panchakarma* treatments, Maharishi Panchakarma does not use all of the 'actions' described in texts, but draws upon those proven most effective in its extensive clinical experience. Since the mid-1980s MAV clinics have administered about 50 000 *panchakarma* treatments around the world. These vary in length from an introductory 3-day treatment, to a more common 7-day treatment, to a 30-day treatment.

In essence, what *panchakarma* amounts to is an integrated sequence of procedures that, together, dislodge impurities from the cells and then flush them from the body. Below we examine the sequence and how it works.

1. *VIRECHANA* (AND *SNEHANA*) – ALSO CALLED HOME PREPARATION

Impurities typically are stored in fat cells, where they can remain for decades. To flush them out, *panchakarma* begins with a form of internal oleation therapy called *snehana*, which takes 4 days. During this time, the individual reduces consumption of oils and fats especially, and of calories in general. He or she then, the first thing every morning, on an empty stomach, drinks melted ghee; other oleated substances such as sesame oil are sometimes used. The amount of ghee is specified by the physician and increases every day. On the fourth day, the individual skips dinner, and takes a hot tub bath, followed by *virechana*, the ingesting of castor oil or other laxatives (again, a dosage specified by the physician). This, of course, leads to purgation over the next 12 hours.

What is happening during *snehana*/*virechana*? Smith & Salerno (1992) suggest the following. First, the reduced ingestion of fats and of calories in general 'favors consumption of body fat stores'. If the fat cells lose fat, the impurities stored within the cells (usually polyaromatic hydrocarbons – PAHs) become more concentrated in the cells by default. Next, the ghee (or other oil) floods the bloodstream with triglycerides. Unlike the triglycerides inside the cells, these circulating ones are free of PAHs, so a concentration gradient is created between the fat inside the cells and the fat outside (the gradient is steeper if in fact the fat cells have lost some of their fat). By the process of osmosis, impurities concentrated within the fat cells flow out into the impurity-free plasma triglycerides produced by the ghee.

Next, these plasma triglycerides, now containing PAHs and other impurities, flow toward the gut. Because one takes increasing amounts of ghee on successive mornings, a good deal of non-circulating ghee is left in the gut, so once again, a concentration gradient is set up between the ghee that has circuited the bloodstream and the impurity-free ghee that remained in the gut. As a result, the impurities picked up by the circulating ghee move by osmosis into the gut. Also, the liver removes some of the impurities from the bloodstream and sends them to be eliminated.

Next, the hot bath increases blood flow to the skin and the underlying adipose tissue; the vasodilation causes lipid-soluble toxins to flow into the blood stream.

Finally, in *virechana*, the castor oil laxative eliminates the toxins and ghee from the intestines. (*Virechana* is also one of the most powerful means of balancing *Pitta dosha*, which is centered in the stomach, liver, and pancreas.)

Snehana and *virechana* are done at home, usually within a few days or a week of beginning *panchakarma* treatment in the clinic. They are referred to collectively as 'home preparation'.

After *virechana*, trained technicians at an MAV health center administer further *panchakarma* treatments in the clinic, on an in- or outpatient basis. These treatments also fall into a sequence. The first group of treatments further stimulates the release of toxins from the cells; the second group causes vasodilation and moves impurities to the organs of elimination; and the third group of treatments then eliminates the toxins from the body. We can call these three groups external oleation, heating, and elimination therapies.

2. EXTERNAL OLEATION THERAPIES

The primary form of stimulation therapy involves massage. There are a few different types of massage, and typically they involve *external* oleation.

Abhyanga (herbalized sesame-oil massage)

This is a warm-oil, full-body massage, administered by two specially trained technicians who work in tandem on both sides of the body (Fig. 10.1). *Abhyanga* normally uses sesame oil; Smith & Salerno (1992) and Salerno & Smith (1991) showed this oil to have anticarcinogenic and, specifically, anti-melanoma and anti-colon cancer effects. Moreover, Japanese researchers have shown sesame oil to contain antioxidants, whose potency is increased when the oil is heated (Fukuda et al 1986, Sugano et al 1990) – and heating is a traditional part of Ayurvedic preparation of the oil.

The oil application procedure itself is designed to stimulate both further release of the toxins from the cells and circulation to the subcutaneous tissues; thus it uses a different type and sequence of strokes than is common in Western massage. The warm sesame oil

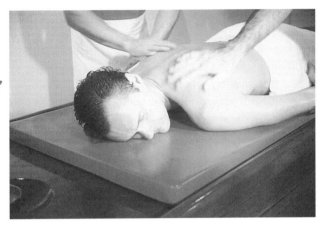

Figure 10.1   A patient receiving *abhyanga*, a full-body massage using warm herbalized sesame oil.

penetrates the pores of the skin, and reaches the subcutaneous adipose tissues, again loosening impurities and toxins. In addition, in Maharishi Panchakarma, the sesame oil is herbalized according to classical Ayurvedic methods to increase its effectiveness. The herbalizing process takes several days and involves as many as 75 different herbs. The *Charaka Samhita* explains the benefits of these medicated oils: 'The effect of taking these oils either internally or externally strengthens the 13 *agnis* [the digestive fires], purifies the intestines, removes *ama* [toxins] from the *dhatus* [bodily tissue] such that the *dhatus* become new, and strengthens the senses, thus preventing aging and giving 100 years of life.'

The oils are concentrated with herbs that penetrate the skin and are metabolized by the whole body. They are said to first remove *ama* (impurities) from the skin, then to penetrate the tissues and remove blockages and *ama* from different aspects of *Vata*, *Pitta*, and *Kapha*.

A wide range of traditional formulas are available; different ones are used in the different stages of *panchakarma* (*abhyanga*, *basti*, etc.). Not everyone receives the same oil for the same treatment. Depending on the predominance of the three *doshas* and the imbalances of the *doshas* (*vikriti*), different formulas are used. Also, certain combinations of herbs have special effects for specific disorders. There are two classes of herbalized oils: *saumya* and *tikshana*.

- *Saumya* oils remove weakness in the body, gently

taking care of disease by purifying one *dhatu* (body tissue) after another.

- *Tikshana* oils penetrate and directly enter the body, causing heat in the blood, improved circulation, and the elimination of impurities. Body type and specific imbalances determine the herbalization chosen.

Udvartana

This massage with a paste made of ground grains cleanses the skin, increases circulation to the subcutaneous tissues, and promotes weight loss.

Garshan

Garshan is massage with raw silk or wool, which creates friction and static electricity on the surface of the skin and increases circulation in the body. It promotes weight loss and clears away clogging impurities that might cause problems such as cellulite.

Nasya

This is a special massage for the head, neck, shoulders, and sinuses. *Nasya* also involves instillation of various herbal drops to cleanse the nasal passages; these are prescribed for different imbalances of the *doshas* and *subdoshas* and for different disorders. During *nasya* treatment, herbal steam is inhaled through the nose, helping to clear excess mucus from the nasal passages and lungs.

The base of the brain is right behind the nasal cavity; thus *nasya* is said to stimulate the base of the brain through its effects on the olfactory nerve endings, bringing greater clarity and balance to the mind, brain, and senses. *Nasya* is said to be helpful in the treatment of all disorders above the clavicle, including those involving the thyroid gland, the sinuses, and the brain and senses. It is often prescribed for headaches.

Shirodhara

In this treatment, a stream of sesame oil is poured over the forehead, balancing *Vata dosha* and *Vata* disorders such as insomnia, anxiety, or worry (Fig. 10.2).

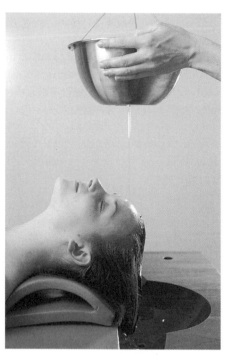

Figure 10.2 A patient receiving *shirodhara*, a treatment in which a stream of sesame oil is poured over the forehead.

Shirodhara is a cooling treatment that settles the mind and profoundly relaxes the central nervous system. It is specifically said to strengthen the *dhatus*, to nourish the nervous system, to increase the glow of the complexion, to increase *ojas* and stability in the mind, and to remove malaise.

Netra Tarpana

This treatment helps remove impurities from the eyes, and includes ghee eyebaths and herbal smoke treatments to cleanse this important organ.

3. 'HEATING' TREATMENTS

Heating treatments dilate the *shrotas* (the channels of the body such as the arteries, veins, and lymph system), allowing the impurities that were loosened through oil massage to be swept away. Heat helps loosen the impurities (*ama*) so they can more easily be broken down and eliminated. The *ama* becomes less solid and begins flowing toward the intestinal tract for elimination. The heating treatments increase circulation of fluids, allowing the impurities to flow easily through the lymphatic and circulatory systems.

All the heating treatments help remove impurities from the musculoskeletal system, where *Vata* and *Kapha dosha* tend to lodge and cause disruption. This is why many people find *panchakarma* helps eliminate aches and pains in the joints, muscles, and bones.

Many different types of heating treatments are used in *panchakarma*, including:

Swedana

In this treatment, one's body is enclosed in a cedar cabinet and surrounded by herbalized steam (the head is not enclosed and is protected from the heat) (Fig. 10.3). The vapors soften and dilate the channels of the body, allowing the impurities to move out. *Swedana* also balances *Vata* and *Kapha dosha*. There are various types of *swedanas*, and various indications and contraindications for its use. Charaka, for example, warns against giving *swedana* to alcoholics, pregnant women, diabetics, and those with certain other types of conditions; he recommends it for constipation, back problems, joint problems, earache, headache, asthma, cough, and many other disorders.

Pizzichilli

In this treatment, gallons of warm oil are poured over the body while it is being massaged. The oil goes deep

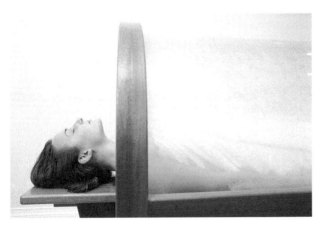

Figure 10.3   A patient receiving *swedana*, a herbalized steam treatment.

into the tissues to balance *Vata dosha*. This is especially helpful for *Vata* problems that are at a deep level of the musculoskeletal system. Warm milk is sometimes used, which is balancing to the skin as well as to *Vata dosha*.

Pinda Swedana

This heating treatment uses boluses, or cloth pouches filled with a precooked mixture of herbs and medicated oils. The technician rubs these hot packs over the body. This is especially helpful in treating musculoskeletal disorders.

4. 'ELIMINATION' THERAPIES

At the end of the treatment each day, after impurities from different parts of the body have been loosened and drawn into the intestinal tract, the patient receives a *basti*. These gentle internal cleansing treatments use either (1) *anu* (warm herbalized oil enemas) or (2) *naruha* (water-based herbal decoctions) to eliminate impurities from the intestinal tract. This is one of the most important aspects of treatment; Ayurvedic texts say that by *basti* alone 50% of illness can be cured.

Because the colon and lower pelvic area is the 'seat' of *Vata dosha*, the *basti* is the most powerful treatment for balancing *Vata dosha*. This is its first purpose; the second is to help eliminate impurities that were dislodged by previous *panchakarma* therapies.

There are two basic kinds of *bastis*:

- Lubricating, balancing, nourishing, strengthening, pacifying.
- Eliminating and reducing.

RESEARCH ON *PANCHAKARMA*

Several studies have examined the effects of *panchakarma*. One looked at how it affects lipid peroxide levels. These relate to an internally created impurity, free radicals. Free radicals have very short lives; but one result of free radicals, lipid peroxides (the damaged fatty molecules that can deteriorate into more free radicals) do have a measurable life span. In fact, lipid peroxide levels in the blood are often used as a measure of overall free radical activity in the body.

In theory, *panchakarma* should reduce lipid peroxide levels. Ghee, as we saw in the diet chapter, is an especially good source of the type of fatty molecules needed to create cell membranes. Sesame oil is a rich source of polyunsaturated fatty acids, and also contains potent free radical scavengers. If cell membranes contain damaged molecules (lipid peroxides and their degenerated descendants), then an influx of ghee and sesame oil could provide intact molecules to replace them.

To study this question, Sharma et al (1993) measured lipid peroxide levels in 31 subjects before, during, and after *panchakarma*. The results were intriguing. During the week of *panchakarma* treatments, the blood level of lipid peroxides actually went up. By 3 months after the treatment, however, the levels were far lower than they had been before treatment. If you sweep a room, dust will fly temporarily, but soon the room is cleaner than before. Apparently, the ghee, sesame oil, and other aspects of *panchakarma* had loosened lipid peroxides from cell membranes and set them free to circulate in the blood. In the weeks after *panchakarma*, the body eliminated these circulating lipid peroxide molecules – and the rate at which new ones were being produced apparently declined.

In addition, *panchakarma* significantly lowered the stress syndrome that creates free radicals. Anxiety, as measured by a standard psychological test, declined markedly.

Moreover, the study showed that *panchakarma* improved several cardiovascular risk factors. VIP (vasoactive intestinal peptide), a neuropeptide which dilates the coronary arteries, rose by 80% after *panchakarma*. HDL (high density lipoprotein) cholesterol, the 'good' (free radical resistant) cholesterol, rose 75% after 3 months in those subjects whose original values were low.

Panchakarma thus seems to be an effective means to rebalance the physiology, and put scavenger and repair mechanisms ahead in their race against free radical damage.

In addition, a study by Schneider et al (1990) looked at the psychological effects of *panchakarma*. 62 subjects were tested before and after a 1- or 2-week Maharishi Panchakarma program with the Profile of Mood States (POMS) and compared to 71 controls participating in a didactic class. The experimental subjects decreased significantly more than the controls in overall distress, anxiety, depression, and fatigue, and increased significantly more than the controls in vigor.

Waldschütz (1988) tested 93 patients before and immediately after Maharishi Panchakarma on various biochemical measures, and 106 subjects before, immediately after, and 6–8 weeks after the treatment using the Freiburger Personality Inventory (FPI). He found significant reductions in total cholesterol and in urea over the 2-week treatment period. On the FPI, he found significant changes on 6 of the 12 scales, including reductions in bodily complaints, irritability, bodily strain, and psychological inhibition, as well as greater emotional stability. After 6 to 8 weeks, the changes persisted. Controls showed no significant changes.

In short, research so far supports the clinical experience of the benefits of *panchakarma*. Further research, we hope, will examine further its detoxification effects, as well as its benefits.

Case study 10.1

S, a 45-year-old woman in good health, began to feel constant exhaustion and depression. A year later, she started to cough incessantly. Four rounds of antibiotics didn't help. She also suffered from severe heartburn, constipation, and pain throughout her body. Her left leg and arm felt numb. After one-and-a-half years of visiting doctors, a pulmonary specialist, using a CAT scan, diagnosed her as having idiopathic pulmonary fibrosis (scarring of the lungs, cause unknown). He recommended that she get a second opinion.

At a tertiary research hospital, her doctor confirmed the diagnosis. He prescribed antacids along with prednisone. These helped, but the symptoms remained.

She then took in-residence *panchakarma* at an MAV clinic. Within a few months, her energy level started to pick up. Since then, she has received three different *panchakarma* treatments. One part of her treatment included *nasya*, which works on the chest, nose, and neck. She was also prescribed an *ama*-reducing diet, which improved her ability to exercise, breathe easily, and avoid the progression of the disease, and a diet to reduce stomach acid and heartburn. She was also prescribed herbal supplements. She learned special breathing techniques (*pranayama*) to exercise her lungs, and the Transcendental Meditation technique.

Within a year, the patient could hold an hour-long conversation without coughing. Her heartburn was gone, without using antacid pills. Her blood pressure was normal, and her HDL had doubled. She could cut back her prednisone from 60 to 10 mg per day.

Case study 10.2

R, a male, age 46, first showed signs of high blood pressure in his late 20s, but paid no attention to it then. By his 43rd year, his pressure had reached 200/100. He was put on medication. The side-effects of the medication, including increased irritability, troubled him. He tried Maharishi Panchakarma as an alternative. Before the treatment, his pressure was 160/90; afterwards, it was 140/80. Also, his irritability had significantly decreased. He repeated the *panchakarma* 4 months later. A few weeks later his blood pressure was 126/68 – in the normal range for the first time in 20 years. This was in spite of his having discontinued medication.

PREPARATION FOR *RASAYANA* THERAPY

One of the main purposes of Maharishi Panchakarma is to prepare the body for *rasayana* therapy (see Chapter 8). Once the *shrotas* (Ch. 5) are clear, the herbs and *rasayanas* can have a much more powerful effect. By analogy, to dye a cloth, first you clean the cloth: Maharishi Panchakarma cleanses the fine fabric of the body, so that *rasayanas* can produce a maximal effect.

MAINTAINING RESULTS AT HOME

The morning routine described in the last chapter can be thought of as a supplement to *panchakarma*, doing something to remove impurities at the beginning of every day. After one has had *panchakarma*, it is a way of consolidating and extending the benefits of the therapy, though by itself it is seldom enough; *panchakarma* is vastly more powerful.

Chapter 9 recommended a daily *abhyanga* (oil massage), taken each morning at home and followed by a warm bath. This self-massage has a similar effect (though on a smaller scale) as the *abhyanga* during *panchakarma*, because it loosens the impurities and clears the channels of the body. *Abhyanga* also settles the nerves through the sense of touch. The warm bath or shower that follows allows the *shrotas* (arteries, veins, lymphatic channels) to dilate and the impurities to flow out, as do the heating treatments of *panchakarma* (e.g. *swedana*).

This simple home routine is an effective way to assist the body in removing waste and impurities, and thus to maintain, or even increase, the benefits of *panchakarma*.

REFERENCES

Ames B N, Profet M, Gold L S 1990a Dietary pesticides (99.99% all natural). Proceedings of the National Academy of Science 87:7777

Ames B N, Profet M, Gold L S 1990b Nature's chemicals and synthetic chemicals: comparative toxicology. Proceedings of the National Academy of Science 87:7782

Bahn A K, Rosenwahlke I, Hermann M, Grover P, Stellman J, O'Leary K 1976 Melanoma after exposure to PCBs. New England Journal of Medicine 295:450

Fukuda Y, Nagata M, Osawa T, Namiki M 1986 Contribution of lignan analogues to antioxidative activity of refined unroasted sesame seed oil. Journal of the American Oil Chemists' Society 63(8):1027–1031

Kahn P C, Gockfeld M, Nygren M et al 1988 Dioxins and dibenofurans in blood and adipose tissues of Agent Orange-exposed Vietnam veterans and matched controls. Journal of the American Medical Association 259(11):1661

Kimbrough R D, Squire R A, Linder R E, Standberg J D, Maotali R J, Burse V W 1975 Induction of liver tumors in Sherman strain female rats by polychlorinated biphenyl Arochlor 1260. Journal of the National Cancer Institute 55L:1453

Kritchevsky D 1985 Influence of dietary fiber on xenobiotics. In: Finlay J W, Schwass D E (eds) Xenobiotic metabolism: nutritional effects. American Chemical Society, Washington DC, p 51

Nigro N D, Bhadrachari N N, Chomchai C 1973 A rat model for studying colonic cancer: effect of cholestyramine on induced tumors. Diseases of Colon and Rectum 16:438–443

Rogan W J, Gladen B C 1992 Neurotoxicology of PCBs and related compounds. Neurotoxicology 13(1):27–35

Rogan W J, Gladen B C, Hung K L et al 1988 Congenital poisoning by polychlorinated biphenyls and their contaminants in Taiwan. Science 241:334

Safe S 1982 Halogenated hydrocarbons in aryl hydrocarbons identified in human tissues. Toxicol Environ Chemistry 5:153

Salerno J W, Smith D E 1991 The use of sesame oil and other vegetable oils in the inhibition of human colon cancer growth in vitro. Anticancer Research 11:209–216

Schnare D W, Ben M, Shields M G 1984 Body burden reductions of PCBs, PBBS and chlorinated pesticides in human subjects. Ambio 13:37

Schnare D W, Denk G, Shields M, Brunton S 1982 Evaluation of a detoxification regimen for fat stored xenobiotics. Medical Hypotheses 9:265

Schneider R H, Cavanaugh K L, Kasture H S et al 1990 Health promotion with a traditional system of natural health care: Maharishi Ayur-Veda. Journal of Social Behavior and Personality 5(3):1–27

Sharma H M, Nidich S, Sands D, Smith D E 1993 Improvement in cardiovascular risk factors through Panchakarma purification procedures. Journal of Research and Education in Indian Medicine 12(4):2–13

Smith D E, Salerno J W 1992 Selective growth inhibition of a human malignant melanoma cell line by sesame oil in vitro. Prostaglandins Leukotrienes and Essential Fatty Acids 46:145–150

Sugano M, Inoue T, Koba K et al 1990 Influence of sesame lignans on various lipid parameters in rats. Agricultural and Biological Chemistry 54(10):2669–2673

Waldschütz R 1988 Influence of Maharishi Ayur-Veda purification treatment on physiological and psychological health. Erfahrungsheilkunde – Acta medica empirica 11:720–729

11

Exercise

Western medicine holds that moderate regular exercise is good for health, and, as far as that goes, Maharishi Ayur-Veda (MAV) agrees. But MAV adds several insights. First, it gives principles for determining the amount and kind of exercise that is best for a given individual. Second, in addition to conventional exercise, MAV provides its own, distinctly different program. Conventional exercise strengthens the muscles and cardiovascular system; MAV exercise does this too, but also aims to make the body highly flexible and, most importantly, to integrate the mind and body.

In this chapter, we examine first conventional, and then MAV exercise.

SOME GUIDELINES FOR CONVENTIONAL EXERCISE

Moderation

Like many valuable practices, exercise has its points of diminishing returns. When jogging was a national fad, thousands of people – some experts say many of the serious joggers – suffered such side-effects as splintered shinbones and broken ankles. And excessive exercise can have a variety of more severe health consequences. Exercise can give strength but it exacts costs if not properly moderated.

While research on exercise gives conflicting results, it appears to support the MAV view that too much exercise can be almost as harmful as too little. Exercise, the ancient Ayurvedic texts say, should be practiced 'daily, in moderation'. What, however, constitutes 'moderation'? If one key to good health is to get neither too little nor too much exercise, how does one determine the right amount? Western experts often suggest exercising between 70% and 85% of maximum heart rate. MAV, by contrast, says that when one starts to sweat profusely, or when breathing begins to be heavy or labored so that one has to breathe through the mouth, that is the time to stop exercising. This amount of exercise, which is understood to be 50% of capacity, is balanced and ideal for health.

If this seems to differ from Western medical advice, it is because MAV wants exercise to accomplish something more than just to strengthen the muscles and cardiovascular system. In MAV, the key to health is maintaining the whole physiology's overall internal balance. Pushing the body near its maximum capacity does strengthen the musculature, and may have localized benefits, but it can cause strain and imbalances in other parts of the body. The system as a whole loses balance, even though some of its parts gain strength.

Exercise and free radicals

The idea of moderation is in accord with recent scientific understandings of exercise. By this view, one reason that exercise is beneficial is that it can increase the number and size of mitochondria – the power generators of the cells – and the activity of their oxidative enzymes (Skinner 1991). The extra mitochondria prepare the body for situations in which it is suddenly required to perform at something like its full capacity. This is valuable because sudden exertion, for those who lack the extra mitochondria, will cause the cells to produce excessive free radicals. A major health benefit of being in shape, then, is that it reduces the amount of free radicals formed during exertion, and might thereby slow the aging process.

But free radicals also give us a reason to not push the upper limits of stamina when exercising. Straining at exercise, which happens if we exercise to 100% or even 80% of capacity, accelerates metabolic processes, which at these levels generate excess free radicals even when one is 'in shape'. The result, as Ayurveda has always said, damages the system as a whole, even if it strengthens one particular muscle group.

50%

For this reason, again, MAV recommends moderation, through exercising to 50% of capacity. By 'capacity' is meant something different from 'maximum pulse rate': capacity is the maximum one can do. For example, if a person can run 6 miles, 50% means running 3 miles daily at the same speed; if one can swim 12 laps, 50% means 6 laps daily. This may seem a small amount to those used to working out, but it is more strengthening than it seems. As one continues to exercise daily, one's capacity will increase. Also, because it does not strain the system, one can exercise every day without damaging oneself, and MAV does recommend exercising daily. By contrast, many challenging exercise programs, which strain the physiology, should be done only three times a week, because the body needs time to recuperate afterwards.

Again, the 50% point is reached when one is perspiring significantly on the forehead or underarms, or when one needs to breathe hard through the mouth. When one exercises, one should choose a pace that leaves one at a degree of exertion just before that 50% point – though the breathing and heart rate should definitely be accelerated. One should maintain that pace until the 50% point is about to be exceeded or until one is starting to become fatigued. At that point, one should stop.

The 50% principle produces an immediate benefit: one feels better when one finishes exercising. Exhaustion during or after exercise is an indication of strain and imbalance. By contrast, exercising to 50% leaves one feeling exhilarated and enlivened, not spent. For that reason, this kind of exercise program is self-reinforcing. One of the disadvantages of overstrenuous exercise is the high dropout rate. Since people tend to not follow through, they lose the long-term benefits of exercise. Because the MAV approach makes exercise enjoyable, natural, and not a strain, people have been more inclined to continue with it daily (this is especially true of middle-aged and older people).

This advice, by the way, does not necessarily apply to professional athletes, who have to work hard to excel at what they do. It does suggest, though, that athletes should take care of themselves in other ways – through the MAV daily routine, *panchakarma*, *rasayanas*, and TM in particular – to help stop unwanted strains or imbalances from accumulating, and to reduce the damage produced by free radicals. Athletes have reported that these programs improve their performance as well as their health.

Individual differences: age and predominant *doshas*

MAV adds another insight to the modern approach, by giving its own guidelines for determining how much and what kind of exercise each individual needs. Two factors have to be taken into account before anyone should start an exercise program. The first factor, familiar to Western medicine, is age. People under 25 should exercise vigorously and regularly. This builds up strength while the body is still growing, strength that will last as the body gets older. People from 25 to 40 should exercise somewhat more moderately, depending on their constitutional type, a factor we discuss below. Finally, people over 40 should be still more moderate. Over the decades, exercise should be increasingly light, though regular – approximately half an hour of exercise daily. This advice is given for several good reasons, but ultimately, the main reason is that *Vata dosha* dominates more and more with age, and exercise increases *Vata dosha*.

The second factor is *prakriti* or predominant *dosha*. Exercise increases *Vata dosha*, the metabolic principle which governs movement in the body, and decreases *Kapha*, the factor that creates weight. Therefore, *Kaphas* – usually larger, slower-moving people, whose bodies have relatively more of the *Kapha* element – need more vigorous exercise, in order to reduce *Kapha* and avoid lethargy and dullness. *Vatas* – usually thin, quick-moving people – should take mild (though daily) exercise, to avoid fatigue, emaciation, and overexcitation. *Pittas* are in the middle: a moderate amount will serve them best. Most people's doshic balance is a mixture, so they should integrate the advice for different *doshas*. This advice will apply more and more as one gets older, but one should start to apply it at age 25.

Specific exercises

To be more specific, *Vata* predominants often find that walking is the daily exercise best suited for them.

Light bicycling or light swimming are suitable too. In general, *Vatas* do best with slow-paced, light exercise that keeps the body in motion for 15 to 20 continuous minutes. *Pitta* predominants enjoy these too, but have more stamina than *Vatas* and will naturally be more vigorous. They also are especially keen on competitive sports. Brisker-paced but moderate exercise that keeps the *Pitta* body in motion for 15 to 20 continuous minutes is best for their daily exercise. Suggested exercises include brisk walking, moderate cross-country skiing, swimming, cycling, weight lifting, tennis, and racketball. *Kaphas* will have the highest capacity and greatest need for exercise. Vigorous exercise that lasts for 15–30 minutes is best. They might try jogging, vigorous bicycling, swimming, cross-country skiing, aerobic workouts, walking, and heavy weight lifting.

Walking is an excellent exercise for almost anyone; *Vatas* can be more moderate with it, while *Kaphas* can walk more briskly and at longer length. But even walking can be overdone, and one should not go for long walks in the heat of the summer sun or in the chill of the winter wind. A comfortable pair of shoes will protect the feet. In hot weather, one might go walking in the early morning. In very cold weather, one might want to take the walk indoors, in a shopping mall or museum, for example, or to substitute an exercise machine, such as a rowing, bicycling, or cross-country skiing machine If one uses a machine, one will get better results with a machine that exercises the lower part of the body, since more of the overall muscle mass is located there. As a general principle, exercises that involve continuous movement, such as walking or bicycling, are more likely to fulfill MAV and Western advice than 'stop and start' sports, like baseball or tennis.

When to exercise

Finally, the time of day when one exercises is considered important. The cycle of the three *doshas* over the course of the day is critical here. MAV considers morning the best time for physical exercise; the *Kapha* period from sunrise to 10 a.m. is preferred, in that exercise counteracts Kaphic tendencies. The *Pitta* period of day, around noon, is not recommended, in that it coincides with the main meal of the day. Also, exercise tends to heat one, and in hot weather midday is especially unsuitable for exercising. Afternoon is acceptable. The evening is not considered a good time for strenuous exercise, since it is too close to bedtime, although a walk after dinner is considered health-promoting. It is better to devote the evening to more relaxing activity. This will be especially important for *Vatas* and for those with sleep problems. This also corresponds with the modern understanding that at night 'the body is less "efficient", has a smaller work capacity and a greater need of oxygen to fulfill this capacity … subjectively, also exercise at night is hardest' (Minors & Waterhouse 1981, p 54; see also Hildebrandt & Engel 1972; Costa et al 1979; Ilmarinen et al 1980).

Seasonal factors also bear on exercise: one needs the least amount of exercise in the very hot weather of summer, and the most in winter and spring, when it counteracts *Kapha*.

When not to exercise

The ideal of daily exercise applies except during an acute illness or, for women, during the monthly period and during pre- and post-partum periods. It is also important not to exercise too near to meal time. After exercise, one should wait at least a half hour before eating. After eating a large meal, one should wait at least 2 hours before exercising (1 hour will do for a snack or light meal) (Box 11.1).

MAV EXERCISE

In addition to its advice regarding conventional exercise, MAV recommends unique exercises which are especially useful for promoting balance and health. It calls them neuromuscular integration (*yoga asanas*) and neurorespiratory integration (*pranayama*) exercises, and, as their names imply, they affect much more than the muscles and cardiovascular system. They help balance the nervous system and breathing, and, most important, integrate the mind and body.

One need not discontinue conventional exercises to do the Ayurvedic ones; the two approaches complement each other. But daily MAV exercises, along with daily brisk walking, serve as a complete exercise program for many people. These exercises are derived

---

Box 11.1   MAV's guidelines on exercise

- In general, exercise to 50% of your capacity. For example, if you can swim 12 laps at most, stop after 6.
- Exercise every day unless you are ill.
- Don't exercise on a full stomach – wait 2 hours after a full meal. Also, after you finish exercising, wait half an hour before eating again.
- Do not strain when you exercise. If you start to breathe heavily through the mouth or start perspiring, cut back for now and then gradually increase the amount of exercise. Your capacity will increase with regular exercise. If you feel invigorated, not fatigued, at the end of your exercise period, you are doing the right amount.
- Exercise during the *Kapha* cycle in the morning (6 a.m. to 10 a.m.) for best results. If you practice meditation, the best time to do most exercises is just after your meditation (except for neuromuscular integration exercises and the *surya namaskara* (sun salutation), which are ideal for settling the mind and body before meditation).
- The correct amount and intensity of exercise depends on age: those under 25 need most, those over 40 need to be more moderate. It also depends on the predominant *dosha*:
  - *Vata*: Slow-paced, light exercise that keeps the body in motion for 15 to 20 continuous minutes is best. Suggested exercises include walking, swimming, yoga exercises, and light bicycling.
  - *Pitta*: Brisker-paced but moderate exercise that keeps your body in motion for 15 to 20 continuous minutes is best. Suggested exercises include brisk walking, moderate cross-country skiing, swimming, cycling, weightlifting, tennis, and racketball.
  - *Kapha*: Vigorous exercise that lasts for 15 to 30 minutes is best. Suggested exercises include jogging, vigorous bicycling, swimming, cross-country skiing, aerobic workouts, walking, and heavy weightlifting.
  - Exercises for all three *doshas*: Walking and neuromuscular and neurorespiratory integration exercises are good for anyone. You can vary the speed and intensity of your walk according to predominant functional *dosha*. *Kaphas* may prefer jogging or aerobic walking, while *Vatas* may prefer a continuous stroll.

Remember that these are only suggestions; one should not feel restricted by these lists.

---

from an aspect of Vedic Science called *yoga*. *Yoga* means 'union' or 'integration,' and its physical exercises are designed to produce integration of mind, body, and breathing.

These exercises also, when done regularly, make the body much more flexible. One of the most common complaints about old age is stiffness: dried out by *Vata*, the joints become stiff and arthritic. Bending over to tie one's shoes, for example, can become almost impossible. In walking one may become slow and stooped over. Regular MAV exercise, done over time, is designed to prevent that, and studies have shown that those who practice it maintain a flexible physiology – a lightness in the limbs – that is characteristic of a more youthful body.

Also, Ayurvedic exercises enliven the *marmas*, 107 vital points in the body just beneath the skin, which are considered to be connecting points between mind and body. Specific *marmas* are said to influence specific organ systems, so each exercise, by enlivening certain *marmas*, is understood to affect certain organs. Enlivening *marmas* is also said to increase balance throughout the body as a whole.

THE THREE KINDS OF MAV EXERCISE

MAV exercise works on three levels – the body, the breath, and the mind. The exercises are practiced daily in a progression from grosser to subtler; one begins with the body (*suryanamaskar* – 'sun salute' – followed by the neuromuscular integration program – *asanas*), then goes to the breathing (the neurorespiratory integration program – *pranayama*) and, finally, the mind (Transcendental Meditation).

These exercises are designed to chip away at blocks of stress (in physical terms, areas of dysfunction) which deposit over the years in the physiology as a result of physical or emotional injuries, worries, and traumas. This stress is said to accumulate most in the spine (and the areas adjacent to it in neck, back, and shoulders) and in the 107 vital points of the body, the *marmas*. The physical and breathing exercises loosen and soften the blocks of stress; the mental techniques are designed to complete the process by dissolving them at their root, the mind-body junction.

In this way, these exercises increase physical and mental flexibility, lightness, vitality, and mental clarity. Below is instruction in *suryanamaskar*; the other two programs require direct instruction.

Suryanamaskar

Suryanamaskar (the 'sun salute') is an exercise which simultaneously integrates the whole physiology – body, mind, and breath. It also strengthens all the major muscle groups of the body. It's an ideal basic exercise program, in conjunction with daily walking.

The *suryanamaskar* is a cycle of 12 positions performed one after the other. You hold all but one of the positions for about 5 seconds, so each cycle takes about a minute. It is a good idea to increase the number of cycles gradually, so as to avoid strain and muscle fatigue. This is especially important if one has not been exercising regularly before. One should stop when one notices heavy breathing or perspiration, or fatigue; at that point one should lie down and rest for a minute or two. With regular performance, one's capacity will increase.

MAV recommends a maximum of 12 cycles in a set. One can do a set of twelve (or less) as often as one wants within reason, but again, one should build up to it gradually. Again, it is better not to exercise at night: the ideal time is first thing in the morning, right after bathing, but any time during the day is suitable. For maximum results, one should do the exercises daily. As with any exercise, it is best not to do it either on a full stomach – wait an hour or two after meals – or right before eating (wait a half hour).

Suryanamaskar involves a specific pattern of breathing. Starting with the second position, on alternate positions inhale and exhale (except for the sixth position. Breathing will be reviewed as we explain each position). One begins to inhale as one starts to move into the second position, and then, once one's lungs are full, one holds the breath until one has finished holding the second position. Then, one starts to exhale as one begins to move into the third position. One holds the breath out until one starts to move into the fourth, where one will begin to inhale.

The 12 positions are as follows:

1. Standing up, with feet close together, place the palms and fingers of the hands together in front of the chest. Gaze forward (5 seconds). Breathe normally (Fig. 11.1).

2. 'Raised arm' position: Raise the hands, which are no longer touching, over the head with palms facing forward. (Do this and all movements without hurry.) Start to inhale as you begin this movement, and once you've inhaled, hold the breath in until you start to move into the next position. Continue to extend the arms till they are slightly behind the head, and lean slightly back from the waist. Gaze up at the ceiling or sky. Hold the position and inhaled breath for 5 seconds (Fig. 11.2).

3. 'Hand to foot' position: As you exhale, lean for-

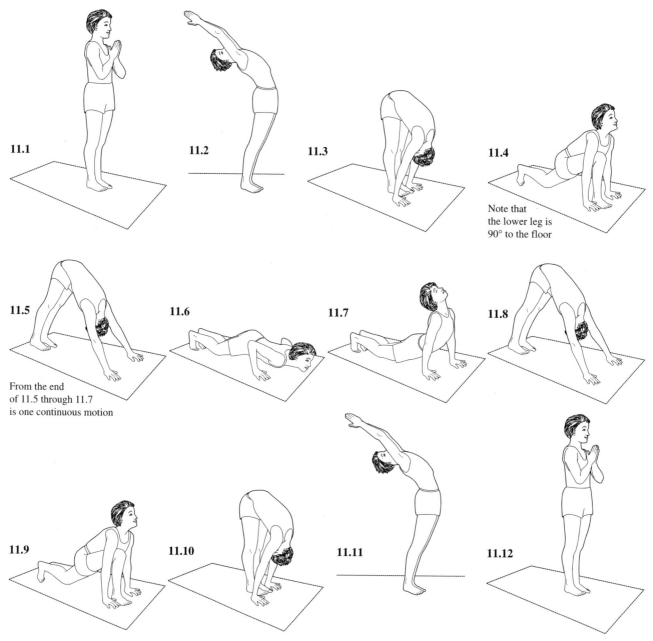

Figure 11.1–11.12 *Suryanamaskar*: the 12 positions.

ward and touch the ground in front of your feet, with hands about shoulder width apart. If you can touch the floor with your palms, that is ideal – but only go as far towards accomplishing that as you can do without strain. Have the head as close to the knees as possible without strain. Keep the knees straight. Only bend as far forward as you can do without pain or discomfort – you'll become more flexible with regular practice.

Hold the position and the exhaled breath for 5 seconds (Fig. 11.3).

4. 'Equestrian' position: Inhaling, keep the hands on the floor at about shoulder width, send the right leg straight back, and bend the left leg at the knee. The left knee goes right beneath the left armpit. The right knee and toes are touching the ground. Arch the back and neck, so that you are gazing up at the ceiling or

sky. Hold the position and the breath for 5 seconds (Fig. 11.4).

5. 'Mountain' position: Exhaling, place the left leg back with the right leg, and simultaneously raise the hips and buttocks so that they are pointing straight up. The knees and back are kept straight. The palms and fingers are on the floor at about shoulder width apart, with the head held in a straight line with the back, right between the arms. If possible, have the feet flat on the floor, but don't strain your leg muscles to accomplish that – just do what you can comfortably. Hold the position and exhalation for 5 seconds (Fig. 11.5).

6. 'Eight limbs' position: Briefly – place the whole weight of the body on the toes and hands, as the chin, chest, and knees lightly touch the floor. The hips are raised so as not to touch the floor. This position is not held, but is passed through briefly. Continue to hold the exhalation from the previous position (Fig. 11.6).

7. 'Cobra' position: Inhaling, keeping the hands in place, straighten the arms, with the knees and toes touching, with the neck and spine arched back and the gaze directed straight up. Hold for 5 seconds (Fig. 11.7).

8. 'Mountain' position: Repeat position 5 – exhaling, simultaneously raise the hips and buttocks so that they are pointing straight up. The knees and back are kept straight. The palms and fingers are on the floor at about shoulder width apart, with the head held in a straight line from the back, right between the arms. The feet are, if you can do it without strain, flat on the floor. Hold the position and exhalation for 5 seconds (Fig. 11.8).

9. 'Equestrian' position: Repeat position 4 – inhaling, keep the hands on the floor at about shoulder width, and bend the left leg at the knee. The left knee goes right beneath the left armpit. The right knee and toes are touching the ground. Arch the back and neck, so that you are gazing up at the ceiling or sky. Hold the position and the breath for 5 seconds (Fig. 11.9).

10. 'Hand to foot' position: Repeat position 3 – exhaling, and straightening your knees, put your full weight back on to your feet as you bend forward at the waist and hips. If you can touch the floor with your palms, that is ideal – otherwise, go as far as you can without strain. Have the head as close to the

knees as possible without strain. Keep the knees straight. Hold the position and the exhaled breath for 5 seconds (Fig. 11.10).

11. 'Raised arm' position: Repeat position 2 – raise the upper half of the body until you are upright again, raising the arms over the head with palms facing forward. (Start to inhale as you begin this movement, and once you have inhaled fully, hold the breath in until you start to move into the next position.) Continue to pull the hands till they are slightly behind the head, and lean slightly back from the waist. Gaze straight up at the ceiling or sky. Hold the position and inhaled breath for 5 seconds (Fig. 11.11).

12. Repeat position 1, but this time exhale and hold breath out for 5 seconds. Stand straight up, with palms and fingers against each other in front of the chest, and the gaze directed forwards (Fig. 11.12).

This completes one cycle.

You should then immediately start the second cycle, by continuing to hold position 12, but breathing as you desire for 5 seconds. This becomes position 1 of the second cycle.

An important point: on alternate cycles, alternate which foot is sent back and which is sent forward in positions 4 and 9, the 'equestrian' position. In our instructions above, the right foot was sent back, and the left sent forward; in the cycle that follows, send the left foot back and the right foot forward. Alternate from cycle to cycle. For this reason, you should do even numbers of cycles: 2, 4, 6, up through a maximum of 12 at a time, rather than 1, 3, or 11. This is to ensure that the muscles are strengthened symmetrically.

After you have completed a set of *suryanamaskars*, lie down on your back and rest for a minute or two.

The neuromuscular integration program

The neuromuscular integration program balances and enlivens the physiology. The program uses exercises known as *asanas*, a Sanskrit word that literally means 'seat', and that indicates great stability, something the exercises are intended to produce.

Each exercise is said to enliven a particular group of *marmas* and each *marma* is said to have a range of influence over specific organs. Also, *asanas* usually extend or flex muscles and muscle groups that in most people sit unused, or at least are rarely stretched. Regular practice of *asanas* is said, therefore, to prevent the musculoskeletal rigidity that can come with age.

There are scores of different *asanas*. Because they each have specific, subtle influences on the body, MAV has neuromuscular integration programs for hundreds of specific diseases. For almost any ailment, an expert in neuromuscular integration can prescribe a specially designed program.

A good deal of scientific research has been conducted on *asanas*. To list just a few studies: Udupa et al (1973) have found *asanas* to result in reduced serum cholesterol level, reduced fasting blood sugar level, increased resistance to physical stress, greater stability of respiratory and cardiovascular functions, and positive changes in urinary metabolites of adrenal steroid hormones and catecholamines. Santha et al (1981) found decreased resting heart rate, increased skin temperature, increased EEG alpha index, reduced blood cholesterol level, reduced beta/alpha lipoprotein ratio, beneficial changes in other enzymes, and increased total serum protein level. Nagendra & Nagarathana (1986), in a prospective study of the effects of *yoga* (and *pranayama*) on bronchial asthma, found improved respiratory function, lower respiration rate, increased chest expansion during inspiration, increased vital capacity, and increased breath holding time. Sahaya et al (1975) found changes in metabolism in muscular tissues, and in intragastric pressure. Udupa et al (1975b) found *asanas* to reduce neuroticism, decrease mental fatigue, improve cognitive performance, improve memory, reduce physical and mental health complaints (including gastrointestinal, neuropsychological, and respiratory symptoms, and anxiety, tension, and feelings of inadequacy), and lower blood levels of acetylcholine and cholinesterase activity.

The neurorespiratory integration program

These breathing exercises are derived from what is traditionally called *pranayama* (literally, 'regulating the breath'). These specific techniques for alternating the breathing between the nostrils are said to create balance in the physiology, improve nervous system functioning, and to benefit many specific organs.

Research on *pranayama* has found it to have such effects as: reductions in bronchial asthma attacks, and general improvement in clinical state and laboratory assessment in 76% of asthma patients (Bhole 1967); increased vital capacity, accelerated adrenocortical functions, decreased blood lipids, and increased total serum proteins (Udupa et al 1975a); and increased breath-holding capacity and lowered pulse rate (Nayar et al 1975).

Research at the Salk Institute for Biological Studies and elsewhere has found that normal breathing is dominated by one nostril, and that periodically (every 25 to 200 minutes) the dominant nostril switches (Werntz et al 1983). Moreover, it found that the two nostrils relate to the opposite hemispheres of the brain, and that brain hemispheric dominance also switches in a periodic rhythm, which is 'tightly coupled' with the nasal cycle (Werntz et al 1983). These studies suggest avenues for exploring scientifically some of the mechanisms through which these breathing exercises work. For example, the Salk Institute researchers found that forced breathing in one nostril increased EEG amplitude in the opposite brain hemisphere (Werntz et al 1987) and improved performance on cognitive tasks associated with the opposite hemisphere (Shannahoff-Khalsa 1991). The authors note that the idea behind these studies all came from ancient yogic texts.

In Ayurvedic terms, these exercises create refinement in the body by working on the most refined aspect of *Vata dosha*, *prana vata*. Since *Vata dosha*, which is responsible for movement in the body, 'leads' the other two *doshas*, *pranayama* settles, balances, and refreshes the whole body. Many people feel that effect when they practice it.

There are many different neurorespiratory integration techniques available for different diseases, body types, and purposes. Below we give a general, preventive technique.

How to do a simple neurorespiratory integration program breathing technique

This exercise should be practiced twice a day for 5 minutes. The ideal time is right before meditation, which will be before breakfast and dinner. Neurorespiratory integration techniques culture the physiology for more refined experiences during meditation.

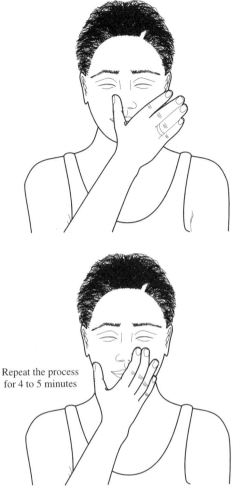

Repeat the process for 4 to 5 minutes

Figure 11.13   Neurorespiratory integration program breathing technique.

When you do the neurorespiratory integration program, sit with the back comfortably upright; it's better not to lounge backwards.

Once again, the exercise integrates the awareness as well as the body, so it is important not to divide the mind by reading, listening to music, or watching TV; in fact, it is better to keep the eyes closed. One should, in any case, let the mind be easy.

Proceed as follows:

1. Sitting upright with eyes closed, take the right thumb to the outside of the right nostril and, pressing gently, close the nostril shut (Fig. 11.13).
2. Breathe out through the left nostril slowly and completely.
3. Noiselessly breathe in through the same nostril and then –
4. Close it with the ring and middle fingers of the right hand by pressing on the outside of the nostril while –
5. Opening the right nostril, by releasing the pressure of the thumb, to breathe out.
6. Breathe out noiselessly, slowly and completely, through the right nostril.
7. Breathe in again through the right nostril in the same way.
8. Repeat the process for five minutes.

CONCLUSION

Exercise is an important part of MAV's approach to creating health. In MAV, exercise is meant not only to strengthen, but also to balance. Thus its advice differs from what is common: conventional exercise is to be done daily to 50% of capacity, rather than three times a week to 80%; the amount and type of exercise you take should be according to your body type and age; and Ayurvedic exercises, performed daily, add profound benefits to those of conventional exercise.

REFERENCES

Bhole M V 1967 Treatment of bronchial asthma by yogic methods. Yoga Mimansa 9(3):33–41
Costa G, Gaffuri E, Perfranceschi G 1979 Re-entrainment of diurnal variation of psychological and physiological performance at the end of a slowly rotated shift system in hospital workers. International Archives of Occupational and Environmental Health 44:165–175
Hildebrandt G, Engel P 1972 The relationship between diurnal variation in psychic and physical performance. In: Colquhon W P (ed) Aspects of human efficiency diurnal rhythm and loss of sleep. English Universities Press, London, pp 231–240
Ilmarinen J, Ilmarinen R, Korhonen O, Nurminen M 1980 Circadian variation of physiological functions related to physical work capacity. Scandinavian Journal of Work, Environment and Health 6(2):112–122
Minors D S, Waterhouse J M 1981 Circadian rhythms in the human. John Wright, Bristol
Nagendra H R, Nagarathana R 1986 An integrated approach of yoga therapy for bronchial asthma: a 3–54 month prospective study. Journal of Asthma 23(3):123–137
Nayar H S, Mathur R M, Sampath K R 1975 Effects of yogic exercises on human physical efficiency. Indian Journal of Medical Research 63(1):1369–1376

Sahaya, Sadasivudu B, Ramananda Yogi et al 1975 Biochemical parameters in normal volunteers before and after Yogic practices. Indian Journal of Medical Research 76 (Supp):144–148

Santha J K, Sridharan S K, Patil M L 1981 Study of some physiological and biochemical parameters in subjects undergoing yogic training. Indian Journal of Medical Research 75:120–124

Shannahoff-Khalsa D S, Boyle M B, Buebel M 1991 The effects of unilateral forced nostril breathing on cognition. International Journal of Neuroscience 57:239–249

Skinner J S 1991 Physiology of exercise and training. In: Strauss R H (ed) Sports medicine. Saunders, Philadelphia, p. 294

Udupa K N, Singh R H, Settiwar R M 1973 Studies of physiological endocrine, metabolic responses to the practice of Yoga in young normal volunteers. Journal of Research in Indian Medicine 6(3):345–353

Udupa K N, Singh R H, Settivar R M 1975a Studies on the effect of some Yogic breathing exercises (Pranayamas) in normal persons. Indian Journal of Medical Research 63(8):1062–1065

Udupa K N, Singh R H, Yadava R A 1975b Certain studies on psychological and biochemical responses to the practice of Hatha Yoga in young normal volunteers. Indian Journal of Medical Research 61(2):237–244

Werntz D A, Bickford R G, Bloom F E, Shannahoff-Khalsa D S 1983 Alternating cerebral hemispheric activity and the lateralization of autonomic nervous function. Human Neurobiology 2:39–43

Werntz D A, Bickford R G, Shannahoff-Khalsa D S 1987 Selective hemispheric stimulation by unilateral forced nostril breathing. Human Neurobiology 6:165–171

12

Gynecology, Obstetrics, and Pediatrics

The approach of Maharishi Ayur-Veda (MAV) to such apparently diverse areas as procreation, prenatal care, and postpartum maternal care can be considered as elements of a single concern: producing the most healthy offspring possible. For those wanting to create not only relatively good health but an ideal state of health, nothing equals beginning at the beginning.

The process of optimizing health can begin even before the beginning. Ayurveda contains a good deal of advice about optimizing the state of both parents' reproductive physiologies before conception. This can include not only treatments to increase fertility and reduce risk factors for miscarriage, but also optimization of the parent's contribution to the reproductive tissues. It can also include advice for women's reproductive physiology, including detailed advice on minimizing menstrual discomforts and disorders. We will begin by reviewing that advice.

MENSTRUATION AND MENSTRUAL DISORDERS

Menstruation's obvious purpose is to let the body slough off the inner lining of the uterus to prepare for another reproductive cycle. According to MAV, menses have other values. They are considered to be one of the body's balancing and healing mechanisms and allow a woman's body to remove accumulated *doshas* on a regular basis.

Menses, by this view, are part of the female body's self-healing system. If a woman knows how to take advantage of them, they can lead to greater balance and better health, removing imbalances and strengthening the system. They also are said to have spiritual value: this is an especially good time for a woman to be somewhat more inward and allow her inner life to grow. If she doesn't handle menses properly, however, they can lead to imbalance and disease.

Dr Balraj Maharshi, one of India's leading *vaidyas* and a major contributor to MAV, says that in his 40 years of medical experience in India he has never seen anything like the number of gynecological disorders common in the West. He attributes this difference to Indian women's greater knowledge of how to care for themselves during menstruation. Western women, he says, typically don't take proper care of themselves during their period. This clinically based hypothesis has, of course, not been tested scientifically, but it may be worth considering.

Below is basic MAV advice on the menstrual cycle, followed by advice on the most common menstrual disorders.

THE MENSTRUAL CYCLE

All three *doshas* are involved in menses, but *Vata* is predominant. *Vata* is responsible for movement, and in particular one of its five aspects, *apana vata*, governs all downward motion in the lower pelvic area. *Apana vata*, therefore, plays a central role in menses. If aggravated, *apana vata* causes aggravation of the other four *Vata* subdoshas. Therefore, most MAV advice regarding menstruation involves pacifying *Vata* in general and *apana* in particular.

Another important consideration reflects the basic understanding that menstruation is a period of purification. During purification procedures, such as *panchakarma*, *Vata* tends to increase because it is taking a more active role in the movement of *doshas*. Therefore, so as not to further aggravate or increase the influence of *Vata*, *Vata*-pacifying measures are recommended, especially proper rest. During *panchakarma*, patients are advised not to undertake strenuous activity, and to have as light a workload as possible. The demands made on the body by menstruation are best met in the same way. Resting helps the body get the maximum benefit, and also helps pacify *Vata*. Hard work during this time has opposite effects.

For perfect health, according to MAV, one must cooperate with the body rather than try to conquer it. When the menstrual cycle comes, it is ideal for a woman to rest for 3 days. Obviously, most women cannot take 3 days off; but if at all possible, they should try to take at least one day off, during the period of the heaviest flow. This may go counter to the economic and social trends of the last 30 years, but ideally society and the marketplace should accommodate women's physiological needs without penalty. Given current realities, most women must compromise, but it can be medically valuable to at least be aware of the ideal situation. A woman can, for example, try to schedule less demanding activities during menses.

When we say that MAV encourages women to rest, we do not mean sleep: daytime sleep is generally not recommended, because it tends to cause obstruction of the *shrotas*, which can interrupt the proper flow of the menses. If a woman feels sleepy, however, she need not fight it; but in this situation she should rest sitting up, and make sure she goes to bed earlier at night.

When a woman is able to rest at home, she should (ideally) engage only in light activities that she enjoys. Reading and quiet, creative activities are ideal. She should avoid heavy work if possible, and refrain from sports, heavy gardening, and strenuous exercise (she can take an easy walk).

During menses, a woman should not practice the daily *abhyanga* (oil massage) or take tub baths. She should substitute a sponge bath or a short, warm shower. (After the menstrual flow stops, she should give her head a warm oil massage, let the oil soak in for 2 hours, and then wash her hair. This will help pacify *Vata*.)

Diet should be light, warm, *Vata*-pacifying, and easy to digest, because the digestive fires are weaker during the period. One should avoid carbonated beverages, which aggravate *Vata*. Especially valuable during menstruation are sweet *lassi* and Ayurvedic buttermilk. One should avoid overeating and minimize foods with a 'heavy' quality, such as red meat, cheese, chocolate, and fried foods. A positive mental attitude is an important element in making the period beneficial.

Research is suggesting that tampons may not be as harmless as they seem (Berkeley et al 1985) – in particular, questions have been raised concerning superabsorbent-sized tampons (Berkley et al 1987, Sun 1982), and those made of synthetic materials (Parsonnet et al 1996). Ayurveda has another concern: tampons are designed to interfere with the free clearance of the menstrual blood; according to Ayurveda, such interference is not health-promoting. Thus, when possible, external absorbers are preferable.

Women who have taken Maharishi Ayur-Veda's advice on all of these points have noticed dramatic improvements in how they feel during menses and afterwards.

MENSTRUAL DISORDERS

MAV has a number of treatments for menstrual problems. Some should be prescribed individually by a trained MAV physician, but many can be implemented easily at home. We will consider first premenstrual problems, and then problems during the period.

During the menstrual period, *doshas* are eliminated; prior to menstruation, these *doshas* accumulate. If the doshas overaccumulate, perhaps owing to previous mishandling of menstruation or to some other form of aggravation of the *doshas* – or if the *apana vata*, which should be moving them out, is weak – these mobilized *doshas* cause various symptoms in the body and the mind. *Kapha* causes swelling and fluid retention; *Pitta* causes heat, hot flashes, eye problems, irritability and anger; *Vata* causes cramps, pain, anxiety, sensitive emotions, and moodiness.

How can one reduce these problems? It depends on the *dosha*. For *Kapha* symptoms, one should avoid day sleep, which aggravates *Kapha*, and follow a *Kapha*-reducing diet. For *Pitta* symptoms, one should follow a *Pitta*-reducing diet. For *Vata*, the most common type, a *Vata*-pacifying routine is ideal.

If a woman has cramps, a hot water bottle (not too hot) helps pacify the *Vata*.

In general, one should take steps to avoid producing *ama*, which clogs the channels of the body. Certain foods tend to have this clogging effect if taken in excess, including cheese, yogurt, and red meat.

In addition, ghee is useful, and aloe vera juice is excellent for *apana vata*. A woman with premenstrual tension should avoid eating eggs, anything fermented (such as vinegar and soy sauce), and very spicy or sour foods, as these aggravate *Pitta*.

For all three types, it is important to have regular bowel movements, for that reduces *Vata* and strengthens *apana vata*.

If premenstrual tension is severe, or if full-scale premenstrual syndrome develops, additional measures are required.

Premenstrual syndrome

Premenstrual syndrome (PMS) can have such extreme psychological effects that it was almost classified by the American Psychiatric Association as a psychiatric syndrome. However, Ayurveda sees it as a build-up of *doshas* in the body. Taking steps to reduce those *doshas* is the basis of effective treatment.

The *doshas* responsible for PMS are *ranjaka pitta* (responsible for blood formation) and *apana vata* (which moves wastes downwards). In the week or two before menstruation, impurities move through the system. Before they are eliminated through the menses, it is as if they have come to the surface. If *apana vata* and *ranjaka pitta* are operating normally, the impurities move downwards and cause no problems. But if these *subdoshas* are malfunctioning, the mobilized impurities can cause the whole range of psychophysiological symptoms that PMS includes.

For that reason, regular *panchakarma*, which removes impurities and pacifies the *doshas*, is very helpful for women with PMS, as are many home treatments. One we often recommend is an aspect of *panchakarma* called *virechana*, described in more detail in Chapter 10. This treatment should be recommended under medical supervision, but, once learned, a woman can use it regularly at home.

Reducing constipation is essential, since constipation aggravates *apana vata*.

Also important is stress reduction. Many women have found TM especially beneficial. Specific MAV herbal supplements can also be helpful.

A *Vata*-reducing diet helps. If the PMS involves anger, then also take measures to reduce *Pitta*, by avoiding very spicy or sour foods such as yogurt, vinegar, and cheese. Also avoid tomatoes, which are potent aggravators of *Pitta*.

Finally, all aspects of the MAV daily routine help establish order and balance, and so are particularly important in combating PMS.

Dysmenorrhea (pain during the period)

Some pain during the monthly period is common, especially when women need to be active and focused. Incapacitating pain is less common, but by no means unheard of. Incapacitating menstrual pain should always be evaluated by a physician, as it may be associated with other medical conditions.

To reduce dysmenorrhea, one should begin by following all the advice given under the menstruation section above. In addition, it helps to establish a regular routine throughout the month – dysmenorrhea often occurs when one has not followed a routine.

Daily *abhyanga* is helpful (though not during the period itself). The woman should emphasize the abdomen, massaging it gently with sesame oil, using a clockwise circular motion, for a few minutes every day. She should follow this with a warm tub soak. This settles and restores order to *apana vata*.

Much of the advice given for PMS is applicable here as well, since *apana vata* is a problem in both cases. Specifically, a procedure that often helps in both situations is *virechana*, performed a week before the period. As we explained in discussing PMS, one should learn *virechana* under medical supervision. Regular *panchakarma* also helps to reduce dysmenorrhea.

One should also avoid cold and astringent foods, such as raw vegetables, ice cream, cold drinks, and raw sprouts, as these aggravate *Vata*. A *Vata*-reducing diet is preferable.

Herbs for dysmenorrhea should be individually prescribed by a trained physician.

PRE- AND POSTNATAL CARE: TAKING CARE OF MOTHER TO TAKE CARE OF BABY

PREGNANCY

Everything a pregnant woman does affects her fetus, sometimes far more than it affects her. It is well known that smoking and drinking can seriously impair the developing fetus, and that caffeine has been implicated too, as have other stimulants, such as over-the-counter cold medicines and any medicines that have not been prescribed by a physician. For the same reason, Ayurveda recommends avoiding very spicy or pungent foods, which are considered too strong for the developing fetus. It is generally recognized that very pungent foods tend to contain more natural teratogens. Garlic, onions, and fenugreek are specifically noted in Ayurveda as having so strong an effect on the body that they could be unsuitable for the fetus. All three have in fact been found in modern research to have significant bodily effects: we have mentioned, for example, science's confirmation of the Ayurvedic understanding that fenugreek lowers blood sugar. Ayurveda also considers fenugreek to be an abortifacient.

Most pregnant women experience some degree of so-called morning sickness and food aversions, as well as food cravings. According to MAV these should in most cases not be considered pathological, but rather expressions of the body's innate intelligence. 'Morning sickness' and food aversions reflect the body's heightened sensitivity to toxins in food that are harmless to adults (including the mother) but can possibly damage the fetus (Profet 1992). Aversions should, within reason, be attended to. If nausea is a severe problem, MAV suggests certain foods as being easy to keep down. A liquid or semi-liquid diet is easily digestible; steamed butternut squash, with a little cardamom; tapioca, boiled milk with a little ghee; fresh peaches; five to ten soaked dates, seeded, then boiled in milk with a little cardamom.

We have all become used to the idea that toxins can damage the developing fetus, which is especially vulnerable to them, and to the dangers posed by nutritional deficiencies during pregnancy. But MAV is also concerned with the opposite: what to ingest to produce the optimal, most positive, most nourishing influence on the fetus. Ingestion here refers not only to food, but also to sensory and emotional input.

Regarding food, pregnant women are advised in most cases to follow a *Vata*- and *Pitta*-pacifying diet: to eat warm, well-cooked, nourishing, wholesome foods, and to avoid rough, heavy, or very spicy ones. Some particularly good foods for pregnant women are milk, ghee, rice, dates, raisins, and almonds, though the diet should be varied and nutritious. The recommendations on digestion in Chapter 7 are more important now than is usually the case; digestion should be as smooth as possible during pregnancy. Of course, pregnant women should not be put on weight-loss or restrictive diets.

Regular light exercise is recommended, but MAV suggests minimizing strenuous exercise, especially anything that can produce sudden jolts to the body or that exhausts the pregnant mother. Ayurveda has always held that mild exercise is better for the mother and baby; modern research is giving some support to this view. For one thing, during pregnancy, blood flow is needed in the uterine area, but exercise causes blood to flow to the extremities. One study found that a 10-minute exercise period reduced uterine blood flow by 13%, and a 40-minute exercise period reduced it by 24% (Lotgering et al 1983). Too much exercise can also cause hyperthermia, which in animal studies has been shown to be potentially teratogenic (Edwards 1986). Theoretically, risks of overexercise by pregnant women could include fetal distress, prematurity, intrauterine growth retardation, and congenital malformations (Artal 1991). A review of published research revealed that women who exercise through pregnancy have smaller babies (Artal et al 1990), and that there is no indication that such women have better pregnancy outcomes in any other way. MAV suggests that a daily half-hour walk is the best exercise for a pregnant woman; mild swimming is also acceptable.

The daily oil massage (*abhyanga*) (Ch. 9) is not practiced by pregnant women, because it loosens impurities from the cells. However, the application of warm sesame oil without a real massage is excellent, since it soothes *Vata dosha*, and helps nourish the physiology and improve the circulation. One exception to the abstention from massage: in the eighth month, mothers should begin oil or ghee massage of the nipples as part of the *abhyanga*. This will help prepare them for breastfeeding. One might use a twisting, pulling motion to simulate a baby's sucking.

The above recommendations benefit the mother's body. As important as that, though, is her mind. Consider what happens to the body when one experiences an emotion. If we become angry, our face flushes and our heart pounds: in Ayurvedic terms, *Pitta dosha* is aggravated. If we feel fear, adrenaline courses through our veins, and our hearts race anxiously: *Vata dosha* is aggravated. In both cases, neurochemicals carry the emotion to every cell in the body, including the cells in the developing fetus. By contrast, joy or love send nourishing chemicals to the fetus.

This leads, then, to the most important Ayurvedic advice for pregnant women: as the song put it, don't worry, be happy. Those around the mother-to-be should do what they can to assist in this. The mother-to-be's state of mind should be pleasant and settled, she should be positive about life and about her pregnancy, and she should be protected, as much as possible, from negativity.

This advice should not become a source of anxiety in itself. Negative emotions do, of course, arise; babies, of course, survive such things; and straining to manufacture a mood is not healthy. But pregnant women should not *entertain* negativity – when they can, they should shift their attention to more positive feelings and circumstances. They should refrain, for example, from watching scary, emotionally intense, or violent movies and TV shows, or from reading frightening or violent books. They should favor uplifting, pleasant, and enjoyable entertainment: Jane Austen is more suitable than Stephen King.

The TM technique, for related reasons, is very helpful during pregnancy – calming, restful, revitalizing, and soothing to the mother and therefore the baby-to-be.

It is recommended that pregnant women avoid feelings of loneliness. Baby showers and similar celebrations are traditional in many cultures for this reason.

MAV suggests, especially for expectant women (and new mothers) with first babies, that they share time with experienced mothers; this is a common, even normal practice in most traditional cultures. Another recommendation is to keep pictures of healthy, happy babies around the house; this practice has a good effect on an expectant mother's psychology.

The husband's role

The husband is of course a less central figure during pregnancy, but he can play the important role of making it easier for the woman to fulfill the above recommendations. The husband should do his best to be sure that his wife is happy. He should also try to help relieve her, as much as possible, of the burden of her responsibilities, for example by helping as much as he can in the daily management of the house.

POSTPARTUM: RECOVERING FROM DELIVERY

According to MAV, among the most important things you can do for a new baby is to strengthen and balance the mother. As a general principle, the baby is more likely to be happy and more settled when its mother feels good. Obviously, this works both ways: a settled baby yields a more rested mother. But improving the mother's condition is sometimes ignored.

The demands on a new mother's body surpass anything in ordinary experience. First, there is the strain of labor and delivery, which comes on top of the exertion of pregnancy; women need months to recover fully. Then there is nursing – a sublime experience, yet one which demands enormous energy. Above all, there is the badly interrupted sleep, and the constant attention a baby needs.

The strain of labor and delivery can be considered in terms of *Vata*'s five subdivisions. *Apana vata* is responsible for downward movement in the lower pelvic region, and in Ayurvedic terms it is this that moves the baby out during labor. This supreme effort aggravates *apana vata*, and in the process throws off all the other *Vatas* in the body. This can cause fatigue, anxiety, weakness, worry, and pain. It also all but puts out the digestive fire, so that digestion usually becomes delicate, and digestive power is at its minimum, adding to the fatigue induced by sleep deprivation and nursing.

Again, MAV holds that everything that happens in the mother's body and emotional life can affect her baby, making it all the more important to attend to the issue of maternal fatigue. Below we give advice for the first 6 weeks after delivery, designed to settle *Vata dosha* and help the body recuperate as quickly and fully as possible.

The mother

Rest

This is often the hardest advice for many new mothers to adopt, because most of us have been so oriented towards activity and achievement, and because society at present is not organized to support it. But the first 6 weeks is held ideally to be a time to forget about career, or even, if at all possible, about shopping and housework. Recovering from the fatigue of childbirth calls for a *thoroughgoing* rest. When the baby sleeps, the new mother, rather than watching TV, beginning a project, or going out to shop, should sleep too. A new mother needs to be flexible, but clear in her priorities: rest should top the list. She should try to delegate all responsibilities. If at all possible, she should arrange for someone else to cook and do her work. For the first 6 weeks, there is an enormous amount of rebuilding, balancing, and strengthening going on inside her body, but, since it is out of sight, one may forget how demanding this process is. For a new mother, the motto might be 'Your work is your rest'.

Obviously, many mothers will not be able to put this fully into practice; there are often jobs and other children to attend to (regarding jobs, obviously, MAV strongly supports maternal leave programs of the greatest length possible). There are, however, other ways of providing maximum rest that mothers might find helpful. Notably, TM allows the mother to gain very deep rest, and to gain it at will, whenever she has 15 or 20 minutes free.

MAV advises that, ideally, new mothers should not go out to public places for the first 3 weeks. This advice sounds stringent, and may be impracticable in many cases, but mothers who have been able to follow it have enjoyed the rest and renewal. They describe it in terms of making the house a cozy, pleasant nest, and enjoying it for the first 3 weeks. If it's warm outside, fresh air and sunshine are good, but it's better to enjoy them from within the home and back yard. If the mother does go out, she should be sure the baby is protected from harsh sunlight, cold drafts, and loud noises.

Many new mothers have found that it aids recovery to limit visits from friends to a few hours in the afternoon, because when guests come one has to be 'on'. A good solution is to establish visiting hours, so that the mother and the house need to be presentable only between 2 and 4 p.m., rather than all day.

One of the best ways of helping the body recover is to go to bed by 9.30 p.m., or as close to that as possible. Even earlier is better, if the mother feels comfortable with that schedule.

Finally, any activity the mother does should be quiet, settled, and easy. This principle is especially applicable in the evening. At night, she should enjoy pleasant, relaxing activity, such as reading stories or singing with her children. Watching TV is not as valuable during this time, as it tends to be excitatory and can disturb the evening's rest.

Diet

After delivery, the digestive fire is delicate, and the new mother should avoid overtaxing it. At the same time, her *Vata* is aggravated. Her diet, therefore, should favor light, liquidy foods, which are easier to digest, and warm foods, which help settle *Vata*. The food should also be nourishing; this will also benefit the nursing baby if she is breastfeeding (which MAV recommends if at all possible).

If the mother is not hungry at breakfast time, she should not eat; but if she is, liquidy, well-cooked farina or cream of rice are very easy to digest, and are nour-

ishing and settling if one adds warm milk, ghee, and brown or raw sugar to taste. This combination settles *Vata dosha*. For lunch, the meal could begin with freshly made soup with a teaspoon of ghee, followed by *Vata*-pacifying food: warm, unctuous, and liquid (Box 12.1). Dinner, too, should favor warm, nourishing, unctuous foods, which settle *Vata*.

Massage

The daily warm sesame oil massage, *abhyanga*, is extremely valuable for the new mother. Unfortunately, most mothers are too tired to massage themselves in the first few weeks. Moreover, the techniques and strokes used in the mother's *abhyanga* are different from those in normal Ayurvedic massages. Daily *abhyanga* by a specially trained Ayurveda technician is

---

Box 12.1 *Vata*-pacifying diet for new mothers

Favor:
- Smaller quantities of food.
- Liquidy, unctuous foods.
- Warm food and drinks (nursing mothers should be sure to take enough liquids).
- Sweet and salty tastes.

1. *Dairy*. Whole milk is good for nursing mothers, at least when warm (and previously boiled) with ghee; they may add raw or brown sugar. Some ginger or cardamom may be added to aid digestion. Take milk separately from lunch or dinner-for example, a cupful mid-morning and mid-afternoon.
2. *Sweeteners*. Raw sugar and honey are preferred; brown sugar is acceptable. Amounts should be reasonable. Minimize chocolate consumption for the moment.
3. *Oils*. Ghee is especially nourishing and settling to new mothers, and also helps with digestion and elimination. Take it in moderate amounts, however: one teaspoon per meal (added to vegetables or rice, for example) and a teaspoon with hot milk before bed and in the morning. Sesame and olive oils are the best vegetable oils during the postpartum period.
4. *Grains*. Rice and wheat are best; barley, corn, millet, buckwheat, rye, and oats are less suitable. Brown rice is too hard for most new mothers to digest; basmati or Texmati rice (which is available at health food and many other stores) are best. Cook it well, with three parts water to one part rice, and a teaspoon of ghee.
5. *Fruits*. Fruits should be sweet, fresh, and fully ripe. They should be taken at room temperature, and eaten after meals. MAV especially recommends sweet fruits such as peaches, avocado, plums, berries, papaya, mango, coconut, and sweet apples. (Sour, tart, or dry fruits are less suitable for the new mother.)
6. *Vegetables*. Beets, carrots, sweet potato, cucumbers, spinach, yellow squash, pumpkin, acorn squash, eggplant, and butternut squash are beneficial. New mothers should

Avoid or reduce:
- Dry foods.
- Raw foods.
- Cold foods and drinks.
- Pungent, bitter, or astringent tastes.
- Food taken straight from the refrigerator.

reduce their intake of peas, green leafy vegetables, broccoli, cabbage, cauliflower, sprouts, white potatoes, and raw vegetables, all of which aggravate *Vata*.
7. *Beans*. Mung beans are the only kind which are both easy to digest and very nourishing; split mung beans cook most quickly and are easiest to digest. They should be cooked in a soup made with five parts water to one part beans until they are totally dissolved and liquidy, and flavored with ghee, which oleates them (otherwise they are too dry); they can be flavored with fresh coriander and a little fresh ginger. One can serve the creamy soup with basmati or white rice. One may find that a full bowl of bean soup is too hard on the digestion and causes some gas; if so, use a smaller quantity of beans. Tofu is also fine, but only if fresh. Other beans tend to aggravate *Vata* and produce gas, and are harder to digest; they are less suitable for new mothers.
8. *Spices*. Fennel, saffron, cinnamon, cardamom, cumin, ginger, salt, clove, mustard seed, and small quantities of black pepper are suitable.
9. *Nuts*. Take only 4–5 nuts per day, preferably ground blanched almonds. The following mixture is considered specifically suitable for new mothers: 4–5 almonds, a small handful of raisins (approximately 15), and 2 teaspoons of flaked coconut.
10. *Meat*. MAV recommends a vegetarian diet for the first month. If the mother craves meat, though, it is best to take it in hot soup form, especially chicken, turkey or seafood soups. One should avoid beef, pork, and lamb.

one of the treatment modalities included in the MAV mother/baby program. During the *abhyanga*, mothers report feeling 'the joy and freedom of being able to let go' – often for the first time in almost a year. They become deeply relaxed and often drift into sleep, something that is always desirable for a new mother.

This last advantage does not apply if the mother gives herself the *abhyanga*, though self-administered *abhyanga* still has great benefits. As soon as the mother feels up to it, she should try to massage herself with warm sesame oil every day. She should pay special attention to her head, feet and hands, but go very lightly over the torso and avoid the breasts. This will be only an approximation of a real 'mother's *abhyanga*', which is a profound and thorough process, but it is still helpful and soothing. After a month or 6 weeks, she will be ready to do the normal daily *abhyanga*. (MAV also recommends massaging the baby at the same time, as discussed below.)

After the *abhyanga*, the mother should soak in a warm tub for 5 or 10 minutes.

The postpartum role of the father

The father's postpartum role is to nurture and protect the mother and child. The mother is so occupied with new demands that she should not have to worry about taking care of herself. The husband can help her by keeping disturbances at a minimum.

In the month and a half after birth, the father should help relieve his wife of household chores, by hiring help, getting a family member to assist, or doing them himself. He should help his wife get plenty of rest, and, most important, he should avoid worry and anger whenever dealing with her, and make every attempt to keep her (and the rest of the family) happy and unperturbed.

Previous children

When a baby is born, it is very important for both father and mother to attend to their older children. The parents should be sure to give them as much attention and love as ever; this is especially important for young children, and requires great attentiveness and sensitivity. One way to help – although this is easier with older children – is to involve the children in the care and nurturing of the new arrival.

Ayurveda considers 4 years the optimum interval between children, from the standpoint both of the children's psychologies and of the mother's physiology.

THE BABY

Caring for mother is also caring for baby, but babies need far more care of their own. The 'how' of this may come naturally at times, but a good deal of it is so new and so unlike anything else the new parent has ever done before that guidance can help. Again, such guidance came routinely in traditional cultures from one's extended family, but nowadays must often be provided by physicians and other experts. Below is some MAV advice on baby care.

The MAV approach to baby care aims to enliven the flow of consciousness between mother and baby, aiding the natural entrainment of their minds and bodies. Many mothers have noted that the advice they received from MAV, such as the daily baby massage, helped strengthen and deepen the growing bond between mother and child.

Feeding and weaning

Mother's milk is the ideal nourishment for a baby. It is not only more natural and hygienic, it is also ideally balanced for the baby's physiology. It also benefits their psychology, contributing to a more secure bonding with the mother. If at all possible, Ayurveda strongly recommends breastfeeding. (MAV treatment can also help with lactation.)

During the breastfeeding stage, the mother should drink lots of milk (warm and previously boiled, and taken between meals), which will help make her own milk more nourishing. If she wishes, she can add sweeteners to the milk, as well as a little cardamom or ginger to help digestion. (We realize that opinions differ on milk today; Ayurveda, however, has always recommended milk for new mothers. If the mother has difficulty digesting milk, she might try the suggestions for milk intolerance given in Chapter 7.)

One should sit up when nursing the baby. This Ayurvedic advice accords with the modern understanding that the baby should be upright while feeding, to avoid constricting the eustacian tubes, which could lead to ear infection.

During the first month, the mother should feed on demand. After that, she should use a 'modified demand' schedule, which tries not to feed more often than every 2 hours. If the baby starts crying within 2 hours of the last feed (timed from the moment that feeding started), it is probably not for food. Mothers may find that a schedule develops naturally – it may well be that the baby needs feeding only every 3 or 4 hours, or it may vary.

MAV considers it ideal to wean the baby at approximately 1 year. Weaning is emotionally easier for the child at this time than at 14 months or later, and easier for the mother's physiology as well. Mothers who have followed this advice after having weaned their previous babies at later ages tell us that weaning at 11 months also cultures a more rapid growth of autonomy and makes the baby feel more self-sufficient. However, this advice is not rigid: maternal intuition may guide the mother to the right weaning time, which may be later in a given baby's case.

Of course, mothers will be introducing the baby to other foods much earlier than 11 months. When the baby starts to cut teeth, and starts to show interest in the parent's food – events which often happen between 4 and 6 months – those are nature's signs that the baby is ready for food that requires more than just sucking, and one can begin supplementing the diet with food other than breast milk. One food should be added at a time, and tried for 3 or 4 days to let the child get used to it and to let the parent notice any possible reaction. One should start with liquids (ideally the broth from either mung bean soup or rice, mixed with one drop of ghee and 1 or 2 grains of salt); then, after a week or two, semi-liquids (try liquidy mung soup, using five parts water to one part beans); then semi-solids ('mushier' mung soup; well-cooked mushy or ground vegetables). After that, if the baby wants more, one should try, perhaps, some stewed sweet fruits. Bananas and sour fruits such as strawberries or grapefruit increase *Kapha*, which can cause congestion, so they shouldn't be given during early infancy. For the same reason, cheese, yogurt, or other milk products should be avoided at this stage. Cow's milk can be added to the diet as the number of nursings per day decreases, usually after 8 months. The milk should be boiled first and allowed to cool to a warm temperature. One can increase the amount given gradually. If the baby finds cow's milk difficult to digest, one could use goat's milk (warm and previously boiled), which is easier to digest than cow's, but less nourishing. Obviously, the parents should avoid foods the baby could choke on, like nuts. Also, they should avoid spicy, hot foods; the infant's system is less able to handle the toxins in these foods than adults are.

When the baby is being weaned, he should eat at the table with the rest of the family; this helps socialize him as well. The mother should in this case breastfeed the baby after he has eaten, and not before.

Miscellaneous points for the first 6 weeks

According to MAV, the most important point in baby care is that the baby should be with the mother. Instead of putting the crib in another room, MAV would have the baby sleep with the parent, if possible in bed with her; many mothers find this is convenient for night nursing. This is recommended especially for the first 6 weeks, though it should be continued for 6 months at least. During the day, the baby should not be left alone for long periods, except perhaps when napping.

In addition, the baby should be kept away from intense sensory stimuli: harsh light, direct wind, cold, and loud sounds. He or she will also be much more sensitive than adults to strong smells – even perfume may be too strong. Ayurveda considers it ideal to keep the baby inside the house for the first 6 weeks, and only to take him or her outside when the weather is mild. He or she should also be kept away from pets. During the first 6 weeks the baby should be kept in a quieter part of the house.

Many mothers have found ghee to be an effective treatment for diaper rash and rashes in general. Ghee is also helpful on the mother's nipples if they become dry or cracked.

The baby's toys should be rounded and soft. They should have no sharp edges, and should not be hairy. They should be attractively colored.

The baby *abhyanga*

Until the umbilical cord falls off, one should gently

sponge-bathe the baby with warm water every day. Afterwards, one should start giving the baby an *abhyanga* (oil massage), followed by a warm bath, once a day. Not only do babies love receiving *abhyangas*, but it benefits them significantly. Research on massage of preterm newborns bears out this claim. For example, even though they received identical diets, premature infants who received massage gained weight significantly faster than those who did not – about 47% more weight gain per day in one study (Field et al 1986, 1987, Rausch 1981, White & LaBarba 1976). Research has also found that premature infants who received massage became more responsive than controls, as measured by the Brazelton Neonatal Behavioral Assessment Scale, and more active. Also, 6 months later, they still showed greater weight gain and better performance on tests of motor and mental ability than those who did not receive massages in early infancy.

Parents of premature babies should of course massage their babies; but MAV is, once again, concerned not only with overcoming deficiencies or problems, but also with optimizing health. That ideally begins at the earliest stages of the child's life. Daily *abhyanga*, then, is done not only to overcome the difficulties of premature birth, but to give normal babies a chance at health as close to ideal as possible.

Traditional Ayurvedic texts say that the daily *abhyanga* relaxes and soothes the baby, allowing him or her to sleep more deeply (parents often report this). It releases muscular tension accumulated over 9 months in the fetal position, and is also said to improve circulation and strengthen the immune system. It is said to strengthen the bond between parent and child, which in itself is beneficial; modern researchers on infant massage have reached similar conclusions (Field 1986). It has a high compliance rate: babies love receiving massage, and parents often find that they enjoy giving it.

It is best to teach this *abhyanga* in person; in this way it is not an intellectual exercise, and the parent quickly gets a feeling for it. It also gives parents confidence to know that they are doing it correctly. Since there are so few trained instructors, and this is so important for children, we will attempt to convey it through the written word, but if you are near an MAV clinic it is better to get personal instruction.

The baby *abhyanga* takes a maximum of half an hour,

including preparation and cleanup. It gives best results if done daily. Although mothers are usually not eager to schedule yet another thing they have to do, this one has intrinsic rewards. The morning is the ideal massage time, but any time, including evening, is fine.

Setting up

The following materials are required:

- Sesame oil, previously cured (see Chapter 9 for instructions), is the oil of choice in most cases. If the baby has rashes or skin problems, coconut oil or ghee may be preferable. Usually, though, sesame is most suitable, except in summer when coconut oil, which is cooling, might be best.
- A very mild, vegetable-oil based or glycerine-based baby soap, which is free of synthetic chemicals and perfumes (available at health food stores).*
- Two large towels, or a large towel and a sheet.
- A baby bath tub (or large sink) full of warm water.
- A rattle for the baby to play with (optional).
- Two pillows, covered with plastic.
- A clean diaper.

The *abhyanga* should be done in a warm room, from which all drafts have been excluded. Wait about a half hour after feeding before starting the *abhyanga*.

Begin by preparing the materials. Warm the oil to about 98°F; you can do this by putting it in a plastic squeeze bottle and placing the bottle in a bowl of hot water.

Now, take the baby and oil to the previously warmed bathroom. Put a pillow on the floor against the bath tub or wall so you can lean against it. Spread a sheet or large towel on the floor, and place strategically around it all the supplies, such as the oil, cleansing mixture, towel for drying the baby, diapers, fresh clothing, etc. Sit

---

*Traditionally, Ayurveda does not consider soap ideal for babies in their first year. Instead, it recommends a special cleansing mixture which is said to nourish the skin. The recipe is: take one-third cup of milk; sift or stir in 3 level teaspoons of besan flour (chickpea flour; be sure to get the 'superfine,' and not merely the 'fine', variety: it should have the consistency of cornstarch – if it is coarse, it is uncomfortable to the baby). Mix the flour into the milk thoroughly; use a whisk to get rid of lumps. Then stir it over a low flame until it becomes thick like a pudding. It should be warm when you use it, and should be made fresh every day. Use it after the baby *abhyanga*, then rinse it off.

down on the towel or sheet, with your back against the pillow, and your legs spread straight out. You will probably want to wear shorts so the oil will not ruin your pant legs. Spread a large towel or sheet over your legs, or put the baby right on your legs if you prefer. Roll up your sleeves, and remove your watch and your rings if they could hurt or scratch your baby. Take the baby's clothes off and place him/her on your outstretched legs, with his/her feet towards your feet.

Now begin the massage, which takes about 7 or 8 minutes.

The massage

1. Have the baby lie down on his or her back on your legs, with the head towards you. Put some warm oil on your hands and begin by gently massaging the top of the head with oil, using a circular motion. Use, to the extent possible, your palms rather than your fingers. Pay particular attention to the soft spot on the head; be gentle with it but don't ignore it. The head massage is said to be good for the nervous system and senses, and to be very calming.

2. Next, gently massage the outer ears (stay away from the ear canals). Replenish the oil on your hands whenever necessary, but use only enough to ensure that the flow of your hands is frictionless. Then do the forehead, using a gentle, straight-across motion. Be sure to keep the oil out of the baby's eyes. Next, go down straight over the cheekbones, using the fingers, and then use the palms, in a circle, on the cheeks, then straight down to the chin. Very gently go over the front and sides of the neck, being careful not to constrict the windpipe and blood vessels.

3. Next massage the torso (remember to re-oil the hands whenever necessary). Begin on the baby's sides at the hips, and pull your hands straight up his or her side, using the palms, continuing up the arms right out to the hands. The arms will stretch out nicely, a relief to the baby after 9 months in the fetal position. Do this three times. This smooth, gentle stroke is used for newborns. After a few weeks, as the baby grows larger and stronger, you can expand the *abhyanga* to include the following: Massage the arms three times each. Start at the shoulders and work to the hands. Use a circular motion on the shoulders, elbows, and wrists, and straight motions on the long bones.

4. Now massage the stomach and legs. Place a pillow (it should be covered with plastic to prevent damage from oil) over your lower leg. Turn the baby 180°, putting his or her head on the pillow and feet towards your stomach. Oil the legs with a flowing stroke, beginning at the upper thigh and going to the toes. Now massage the stomach slowly, in a clockwise circular motion; repeat three times – this is said to be good for digestion. Then return to the legs, using the same motion as before, this time going down the legs three times.

5. Then, using your thumbs, massage the inner thighs in a circular motion three times each. This area is usually constricted owing to diaper wear and it is good to give it special attention to increase circulation. Then again, using the palm, massage each leg, one at a time; use a circular motion on the hips, straight on the thighs, circle on the knees, straight on the calf. Then do the feet – Ayurveda recommends paying special attention to them.

6. Now massage the back. If you do not have a towel or sheet over your legs, you can place the baby's face down with the head towards your feet. If you have a towel over the legs, though, he or she might have trouble breathing in that position, so in that case prop him or her up with one hand under the front torso (the back is facing up) while you massage with your other hand. The back is the most important part to massage; out of the 6 to 8 minutes needed for the whole massage, 3 minutes should be spent on the back. Gently use your full hand to move up and down the back, with emphasis on the up stroke. Use a circular motion on each buttock.

Cleaning up

When cleaning the oil off the baby, you can use a towel to help turn and pick him or her up. Soap or just water can be used for cleaning – you might use soap on alternate days. If you are using the milk/flour cleansing mixture, which is the best option, make sure that it is warm, and spread it liberally all over the body *before* putting the baby in the tub. Do this gently but quickly; because the lotion isn't oil-based, it will cool off fast. Bathe the baby in comfortably *warm* (not cool or room temperature) water. Keep his or her head out of the water with one hand, and remove all the soap or cleansing mixture with the other. Rinse the head well with your free hand, still keeping the head out of the water. When you bathe the baby, be sure to remove any bits of lint or cleansing mixture from the creases on the body.

Finally, dry the baby gently and thoroughly, especially the head. In the warm air, after you have towel-dried, let your baby 'air dry' a little more, and do some simple exercises with him/her. Babies enjoy these exercises, and they are good for digestion and neuro-muscular integration. Each exercise should be done three times, with the baby lying on his or her back:

1. Gently, bending the legs from the hip, push the knees towards the stomach (the legs are bent at the knees).
2. Gently, bending from the hip, lift the legs straight up in the air.
3. With the legs extended straight, cross one leg over the other. Then reverse.
4. Lift the right leg towards the left arm, crossing it over the stomach. Repeat with the left leg and right arm.
5. Spread the arms all the way out, and cross them over the chest.

Dress the baby in fresh, clean, loose clothing and let him or her rest; often babies are so relaxed that they sleep after their *abhyangas*.

Other tips

- A rattle to play with will help keep the baby entertained during his massage.
- If the baby is in the habit of using a pacifier, it is good to have one on hand.

As the baby grows to be a toddler, parents should keep a fun, creative approach to the *abhyanga*. The child can sit or stand; parents become expert at oiling a moving target. Most toddlers love a tub bath; as the child stands by the tub eagerly watching it fill, the parent can give a quick massage as the toddler supports him or herself on the tub.

HEALTH ADVICE FOR TODDLERS AND OLDER CHILDREN

The standard medical view is that children get sick more often than adults because their immune systems are untested and are being exposed to viruses for the first time. When they do come in contact with viruses and upper respiratory infections – usually in the preschool and kindergarten years – they easily fall sick. Later in life, having developed a resistance to these diseases, they become ill less often.

However valid this may be, MAV is centered around the ideal of fostering maximum immune strength, and this can apply to children. We can help keep children healthy through diet and routine.

If congestion is a problem

When pediatricians train in MAV, the question they most often ask is: 'What can you do for congestion?' Congestion, in the form of runny noses, coughs, recurrent colds, and ear infections, is the most common childhood syndrome.

This is because mucus is the waste product of *Kapha*, and childhood is the most *Kapha*-dominated period of life. As mentioned in Chapter 5, different *doshas* predominate during different periods of life. During the growing years, as the physical structure of the child's body is forming, *Kapha dosha* is more active than the other doshas. *Kapha* is slow, heavy, sticky, firm, and strong, and its proper functioning is essential for the body to grow. If *Kapha* becomes imbalanced, its heavy and sticky qualities can slow digestion and produce excess mucus.

Although a child's individual doshic make-up will come into play, an imbalance in *Kapha dosha* is most often the cause of childhood disease, including the colds, flu, asthma, and sore throats that are so common. With changes in diet and routine, we can take steps to keep *Kapha dosha* balanced and thus greatly reduce childhood illnesses.

In treating congestion, MAV's primary recommendation is in diet. If children have frequent colds and runny noses, have them avoid cold foods and drinks. They should also avoid yogurt, cheese, red meat, ice cream, peanuts, bananas, and sweets (try fresh or dried fruits as a substitute for candy). Sour foods should not be taken in excess, either.

In addition, it is important to keep the child's head, neck, and ears covered when the weather is cold or windy. If a child has a cold or other congestive ailment,

---

Case study 12.1

A, aged 4, caught a cold every 6 weeks; within a couple of days, it usually turned into bronchitis. Twice the bronchitis had turned into pneumonia, and twice, also, his parents had to rush him to the emergency room for an asthma attack. Even when he wasn't sick, he usually had a runny nose and congestion that gave his voice a nasal drone. Antibiotics and other standard treatments were ineffective.

When he was brought to an MAV clinic, we put him on a *Kapha*-reducing diet, and added some *Kapha*-reducing elements to his daily routine. This produced an immediate change. He has since then caught very few colds and the colds he has caught went away quickly. He has not needed antibiotics in the 4 years since then and has had no allergies and almost no asthma.

---

he should bathe less than once a day and wash his hair once a week or so. Discontinue *abhyanga* when there is a fever or congestion. The parent can, however, warm some sesame oil, add salt, and massage the child's chest with it, then cover the chest with a warm cloth.

Also, one can use a paste made of a quarter teaspoon of turmeric and 1 teaspoon of honey mixed well together. Children can take this orally twice a day. It can be used for chronic sinusitis as well as for acute congestion.

Obviously, if the cough, cold, or other mucus condition continues for a long time, is severe, or is accompanied by a high fever, parents should consult a physician. Earaches should always be brought to a physician's attention.

General advice for children's health

Much of the advice given in this book regarding diet, exercise, constitutional type, and so forth must be modified when applied to children. The advice given below is meant to supplement, not replace, regular pediatric care.

1. MAV recommends continuing the daily *abhyanga* after babyhood. *Abhyanga* has all the profound benefits for young children that it does for babies and for adults. A daily sesame oil massage, especially on the head and the soles of the feet, is said to help the development of all the tissues. It seems to smooth out psychological upsets, like anger or frequent nightmares. Many parents report that their children become sick less frequently. Use the instructions given in Chapter 9.

This is easier if one makes massage a routine from infancy. Once children are 6 or 7, parents have a harder time getting them to start (though it is usually easy to win them over to the nightly foot massage); but they genuinely like the *abhyanga* when it has been made part of their routine.

Children often enjoy receiving a nightly foot massage, which helps them sleep more soundly. It stimulates *marma* points for sound sleep, and often helps reduce frequent awakening. One parent says, 'I massage my daughter's feet every night before she goes to bed. If I forget, she comes to get me. She sleeps better and seems healthier.'

2. Outdoor games and exercise are good for the growing child's body and mind. Children should exercise as much as they like. Easy calisthenics and neuromuscular integration exercises, such as the *suryanamaskar* (Ch. 11) are also beneficial.

3. Children need more sleep than adults, of course, but MAV believes that they will derive more benefit from their sleep if they get it earlier at night rather than later in the morning. Ayurveda recommends a bedtime of 8.30 (or earlier) for school-age children. We realize that many parents keep their children up later nowadays, partly because the parents' long work schedules do not allow them to see their children until late at night. The cost – children who doze through class at school the next day, and whose growth process may be affected by sleep deprivation – is unacceptable.

4. Children's bodies are changing so quickly that it is often difficult to determine their true predominant functional *dosha*. It is best not to pigeonhole children with labels like 'she's a *Pitta*' or 'he's a *Kapha*', both because they are changing so rapidly and because stereotyping is generally to be avoided with children.

5. Many of the dietary rules given in this book do not apply to children. For example, between-meal snacking is normal for children; they often need the extra food, since their bodies are growing rapidly.

They should, however, snack on healthy, balanced foods rather than junk food. In a natural setting, the sweet tooth, a universal among children, is essentially a craving for sweet fruit, which is of course healthy. In our unnatural environment, Madison Avenue and other cultural influences can start to divert that natural 'wisdom of the body' away from healthful and toward unhealthful cravings. Parents should use common sense in handling this.

A routine for daily meals is important. The whole family should sit together at the evening meal every day. If it is at all possible to arrange to eat lunch and breakfast together, this makes a real difference for them, too. According to MAV, children feel more secure and happy when they eat with their parents, which means that the food they eat has a healthier effect.

Anthropologist Lionel Tiger, who has studied eating habits around the world, says that in many cultures 'the role of food is to make people feel good. It validates the importance of the family and offers some sense of continuity'. One result of the tighter family unit, Ayurveda would predict, is better health, since the children are happier.

Also, children should not be put on *Vata-*, *Pitta-*, or *Kapha*-balancing diets. Their physiologies are changing so rapidly that what suits them one day might not the next. A trained MAV doctor may well put a child with a particular health problem on a specific diet, but this is a special medical case.

MAV advises against forcing any amount of food on children. They should be allowed to eat as much or as little as they want at a meal, rather than either 'clean the plate' or control their appetites. As long as the food we serve is freshly prepared, wholesome, and delicious, children's palates are usually trustworthy (though sometimes they are fooled by sweet snacks before mealtime). Children's food aversions may reflect innate mechanisms designed to protect them from toxins that would not bother adults.

While children should eat what they like, some foods are good staples for most children. These include:

- Cow's milk, which helps nourish all the tissues, especially, according to Ayurvedic tradition, the nervous system. The milk should be taken warm and previously boiled. Ancient Ayurvedic tradition emphasized milk's value for children. If a child has problems with milk, such as allergies or intolerance, one should follow the advice given in Chapter 7 on milk intolerance.
- Dried fruits, especially dates, figs, and raisins (best soaked overnight before eating).
- Nuts, especially almonds, coconut, and walnuts, are good, though parents should wait until the children's molars have grown in so they can chew the nuts; before then, children can choke on them.
- Puffed cereals, such as puffed rice and wheat.

Parents should not rely on these foods only: children should have a balanced, varied diet, so that they get all the different kinds of nutrients they need.

MAV also offers a good deal of advice regarding childrearing and education, but these go beyond the scope of the present book.

REFERENCES

Artal R 1991 Exercise during pregnancy. In: Strauss R H (ed) Sports medicine, 2nd edn. Saunders, Philadelphia, pp 509–511

Artal R, Wiswell A R, Drinkwater B (eds) 1990 Exercise in pregnancy, 2nd edn. Williams & Wilkins, Baltimore, pp 213–225

Berkeley A S, Micha J P, Freedman K S, Hirsch J C 1985 The potential of digitally inserted tampons to induce vaginal lesions. Obstetrics and Gynecology 66(1):31–35

Berkley S F, Hightower A W, Broome C V, Reingold A L 1987 The relationship of tampon characteristics to menstrual toxic shock syndrome. Journal of the American Medical Association, 258(7):917–920

Edwards M J 1986 Hyperthermia as a teratogen. Teratogenesis Carcinog Mutagen 6:563–582

Field T 1986 Interventions for premature infants. Journal of Pediatrics 109(1):183–191

Field T, Scafidi F, Schanberg S 1987 Massage of preterm newborns to improve growth and development. Pediatric Nursing 13(6):385–387

Field T, Shanberg S, Scafidi F et al 1986 Tactile/kinesthetic stimulation effects on preterm neonates. Pediatrics 77(5):654–658

Lotgering F K, Gilbert R D, Longo L D 1983 Exercise response in pregnant sheep: oxygen consumption, uterine blood flow and blood volume. Journal of Applied Physiology 55:834–841

Parsonnet J, Modern P A, Giacobbe K D 1996 Effect of tampon composition on production of toxic shock syndrome toxin-1 by Staphylococcus aureus in vitro. Journal of Infectious Disease 173(1):98–103

Profet M 1992 Pregnancy sickness as adaptation: a deterrent to maternal ingestion of teratogens. In: Barkow J H, Cosmides L, Tooby J (eds), The adapted mind. Oxford University Press, New York, pp 327–366

Rausch P B 1981 Effects of tactile and kinesthetic stimulation on premature infants. Journal of Obstetric and Gynecological Neonatal Nursing 10:34

Sun M 1982 Use of 'Super Plus' tampons discouraged. Science 216:1300

White J, LaBarba R 1976 The effects of tactile and kinesthetic stimulation on neonatal development in the premature infant. Developmental Psychology 9:569

13

Maharishi's Vedic Approach to Health

The approaches covered in previous chapters, together with those covered below, are referred to collectively as Maharishi's Vedic Approach to Health. The Vedic Approach to Health, according to Maharishi, 're-establish[es] balance between the body and its own inner intelligence through Vedic Knowledge and its application'. Vedic Knowledge, Maharishi continues, is 'the knowledge of Natural Law...the knowledge of the impulses of intelligence that constitute the structure of the physiology, regulate its functioning, and express, transform, and expand consciousness in its varying degrees of expression into the material structure of the physiology' (Maharishi Mahesh Yogi 1995).

Maharishi's Vedic Approach to Health holds that

there is an inseparable, very intimate relationship between the unmanifest field of consciousness and all the manifest levels of the physiology: that is why Maharishi's Vedic Approach to Health handles the field of health primarily from the most basic area of health – the field of consciousness – through the natural approach of consciousness, Transcendental Meditation.... It also handles health from the more expressed levels of health, the fields of physiology, behavior, and environment, through natural daily and seasonal routines; healthy, balanced diet; suitable exercise; and herbal preparations.... It also handles health from the field of knowledge – from knowledge of balance – and the knowledge of the inseparable connection between consciousness and its expression, the physiology.

This chapter will touch upon some of the other modalities involved. These involve, among other things, the senses and the environment (from the immediate to the largest environment). There are also some important additional applications of technologies of consciousness; we will end the chapter by discussing them.

THE SENSES

The senses (in Sanskrit, *indriyas*) are, according to Vedic thought, manifestations of consciousness. They are grosser (in the sense of more 'manifest') manifestations than mind, intellect, or ego. They project into the world and at the same time bring in information from the manifest world; that information can affect the balance of the *doshas* and *dhatus*, and thus affect health.

In modern terms, we can see another health impact of the senses. Every sense has a direct channel to the brain and, through the limbic system and other avenues, a consequent effect on the whole physiology.

Maharishi Ayur-Veda (MAV) has modalities that work through each of the senses. Of all the senses, it holds, sound has the most dramatic effect.

Sound

The idea that music and other sounds can affect health is hardly novel. The ancient Greeks, Persians, and Hebrews used music systematically as therapy, and the idea of music influencing the body engaged some inquiring Renaissance minds. In our century, this idea fell out of favor, but in the last 30 years has been coming into its own. Music therapy has emerged as a rational discipline. Research has shown that music affects the growth of plants, and a variety of studies have shown it to have significant effects on the human physiology and psychology.

Investigations have shown that music has many effects on the human body. One study demonstrated that music can change pulse rate, circulation, and blood pressure (McClelland, 1979). Depending on the type of music played, there can be an increase or decrease in metabolism, internal secretions related to metabolic change, muscular energy, and respiration rate (McClelland 1979). One study showed specifically that soothing music decreases oxygen consumption and basal metabolic rate, while exciting music increases both (Cook, 1986). Widespread effects in the body have been demonstrated by another study which showed that different types of music have different effects on gastric motility, electrical conductivity of the skin, pupillary dilation, and muscle contraction (Bruya & Severtsen 1984).

Music has been utilized specifically as a treatment.

A large number of studies have revealed that music can help alleviate acute pain (Cook 1986, Munro & Mount 1978, Owens & Ehrenreich 1991, O'Sullivan 1991, Cook 1981). In fact, music has decreased the need for pain medication and sedatives by as much as 30% (Owens & Ehrenreich 1991, Cook 1986). Music is now used on a regular basis in the delivery room at the University of Kansas Medical Center in Kansas City, where it routinely lowers the amount of anesthesia needed and shortens the labor period (Cook 1981).

Vibrations among the molecules

Recent research has provided a molecular-level explanation for the effect of music – and all types of sound – on the functioning of cells. Cells, subcellular components, and molecules all exhibit characteristic vibrational patterns. DNA structures containing G-C base pairs, for instance, vibrate at a higher frequency than those containing A-T base pairs (Chou 1984). Proteins have been measured with specific vibrational frequencies registering 1 trillion oscillations per second and higher (Chou 1983). These vibrations have functional importance. Vibrations of the myoglobin molecule, for example, encourage the movement of oxygen molecules in and out of the molecular structure. Structural vibrations in enzymes also appear to be important at the active site, where substrate molecules are joined or sundered (Karplus & McCammon 1986, Sitter et al 1985).

Throughout the cell and extending into the extracellular spaces is a skeletal structure which also has characteristic vibrations. In the nucleus, this semi-rigid maze is known as the nuclear matrix. In the cytoplasm, a similar web-like structure is called the cytoskeleton. Outside the cell, it is known as the extracellular matrix. All three components of this matrix are interconnected, and maintain constant vibrational activity.

The rapid vibrations of this system have mechanical effects in the cell. When molecules such as messenger RNA move in and out of the nucleus, they appear to move down lines of this matrix system, guided by the direction of matrix fibers and motivated by their vibrational energy (Xing & Lawrence 1989). Some researchers believe that fluctuations in the vibrational rate moving down the matrix fibers act as a communication system. Even signals from outside the cell can be transmitted through the connecting matrix all the way to the DNA (Pienta & Coffey 1991). Recent studies have also shown that variations in vibrational frequency correlate with various types of cell growth (Myrdal & Auersperg 1986). Cancer cells have a vibrational pattern distinct from all normal cells (Partin et al 1988, Mohler et al 1987).

In view of these findings, it is not unreasonable to consider the possibility that every cell in the body may respond to changes in vibrational frequency coming from the outside environment. When music shows its charm to 'soothe a savage beast', it may do so by altering the vibrational patterns in each cell's cellular matrix and DNA.

Music in MAV

These recent investigations help explain why sounds of different types play a central role in MAV. First, the external vibrations produced by music in the environment almost certainly alter inner vibrations at the molecular level. Second, the melody and rhythmic structure of music is yet another experience to be metabolized through the limbic system, transforming it into a waterfall of neurochemicals and hormones that regenerate the body. Research studies have shown that different types of music have different effects – and masters of the Ayurvedic tradition, with sensibilities refined by years of meditation, have conducted a thorough study of these effects of sound on consciousness. The result is a varied pharmacopeia of music and other uses of sound.

Gandharva Veda. The best known of these is *Gandharva Veda*, the traditional classical music of India. *Gandharva Veda* originated thousands of years ago, and even today its basic principles underlie the long and beautiful improvisations by its master musicians.

The *doshas* can be aggravated or balanced by varying melodies and rhythms. *Gandharva Veda* is precisely calculated to have a positive effect on *dosha* balance. In fact, the classical Ayurvedic texts list precise times of the day for the playing of different *ragas*, or melodies. One *raga* helps create energy and dynamism for activity during the day, another creates restfulness after the evening meal. The music that is right at dawn does not have an ideal effect at noon or midnight.

MAV emphasizes the importance of these natural cycles of the day and season (Ch. 9). Listening to the right *raga* at the right time is said to smooth the natural transitions and attune the body and mind to the circadian cycle. Also, specific *ragas* are prescribed to balance specific *doshas*.

Primordial sound

Research has demonstrated that different sounds produce different effects on the physiology. MAV asserts that particular sounds – primordial sounds – have the most positive effect on body and mind. The pronunciation, melody, and rhythmic pattern of these sounds are said to have been preserved as the basic source material of the Vedic tradition – in the Ṛk Veda and three companion collections, *Sama Veda*, *Yajur Veda*, and *Atharva Veda*. According to MAV, the sound patterns preserved in these collections reflect the primordial vibrations at the basis of nature.

In Chapter 2, we discussed the unified field as the field of pure consciousness, the basis of knower, process of observation, and the observed (respectively *rishi*, *devata*, and *chhandas*). Vedic Science further explains that these three aspects are involved in constant self-referral interaction within the unified field prior to its manifestation. These self-referral interactions produce intricate patterns of vibrations, which are the fundamental frequencies said to be at the basis of the physical structure of the universe; we might refer to them as laws of nature. Vedic Science adds the idea that these vibrations can be cognized *directly* within the purified consciousness of enlightened people. Within the field of pure intelligence, the most fundamental vibrations or patterns are heard as primordial sound. This is said to be the deepest level of direct intuition of subjective knowledge.

Once cognized by enlightened sages, these primordial sounds are said to be capable of being brought out onto the level of human speech. Vedic *pandits* – trained experts in Vedic knowledge – memorize these sequences and pass them down from generation to generation. According to MAV, people who listen to these primordial sounds enliven the basic frequencies within their own consciousness. The individual awareness is brought in tune with the first fluctuations of the laws of nature. Because the unified field of natural law is a field of supersymmetry, of perfect balance,

Maharishi maintains that this experience brings increased balance to the psychophysiology. During this experience, both mind and body metabolize the most basic laws of nature.

He also maintains that the various branches of the Vedic literature are associated with specific laws of nature that give rise to specific aspects of the physiology. Hearing a branch of the Vedic literature is said to balance that aspect of the physiology associated with those laws of nature. This is one application of an idea mentioned in Chapter 2: that there are 40 basic types of modes of vibration of the unified field; that these modes of vibration lie, in a sense, at the root of natural law, including the human physiology; that these can be directly experienced by a suitably refined human nervous system; and that these sounds are recorded in 40 branches of the Vedic literature. The neurophysiologist Tony Nader has found astonishingly detailed, precise correspondences between the branches of the Vedic literature and those of the human physiology (Nader 1995). This idea has many potential implications for both the prevention and treatment of disease; the use of primordial sounds is an obvious one.

Research on primordial sounds. At Ohio State, Dr Sharma and colleagues tested the effects of primordial sounds on established cancer cell lines in laboratory cultures. Five types of cancer cells were tested (lung, colon, brain, breast, and skin), along with one normal fibroblast cell line. In this type of culture, both cancer cells and fibroblast cells ordinarily grow rapidly (the fibroblast cells multiply much more rapidly in cell culture than they do in the human body).

For one set of cell lines, primordial sounds were played – particular selections from *Sama Veda*. For the other set of cell lines, contrasting sounds were chosen – hard rock music played by the band AC/DC. Control cells were grown in an incubator in which no music was played.

The results were striking (Sharma et al 1996). Primordial sounds significantly decreased the average growth in all cell lines. The results were so marked that the chance of coincidence was less than 5 in 1000. In the presence of hard rock music, the effect went the other way: growth of the cell lines was significantly increased (with a chance of coincidence of less than 3 in 100 across all cell lines). The decrease in growth of both cancer cells and normal fibroblasts with *Sama*

Veda is consistent with a balancing effect more in tune with the natural laws of the body. This was a pilot study, and more work is needed, but in this area as in many others the effectiveness of MAV received initial confirmation.

Aroma therapy

MAV also makes use of each of the other four senses. Touch is used above all in massage (Chs 9 and 10), and taste in food choice. As for smell, this too can be expected to have a profound significance. Olfactory cells in the nose are connected to the hypothalamus. At the same time, the message of a particular aroma is carried to the limbic area of the brain surrounding the hypothalamus, which processes emotions, and to the hippocampus, an area of the brain responsible for memory (which is why certain aromas trigger such vivid memories). In Chapter 4, we called this a system for metabolizing experience; and the sense of smell is hard-wired into it.

MAV has modalities that affect every one of the senses, including smell, and uses a wide range of aromas – usually floral or herbal essences – precisely calibrated to pacify specific *subdoshas* or *doshas*.

Regarding sight, a system of color therapy is used to pacify the *doshas*.

THE ENVIRONMENT
Maharishi Jyotish

Quantum physics has discovered that all of nature is deeply interconnected. From one end of the universe to the other, all protons and electrons are simply fluctuations in the unbounded, unified field of pure intelligence. Einstein's theory of relativity showed that space and time are parts of one continuum – space-time. In relativity theory, moreover, measurements of the 'objective' space-time continuum are inseparably linked to the state of the observer (the subject, the knower).

Quantum mechanical investigations have shown the same deep relationship of subject and object, observer and observed (Ch. 2). Recent investigations have also demonstrated that any two subatomic 'particles', once they have interacted, are permanently and instantaneously connected across even an infinite distance. If you use an electromagnetic field to flip one particle over, the other will flip at the same time, no matter how far away, and with no material connection between the two. To many physicists, these deep inter-connections seem a central element of physical creation. Nothing exists on its own, not even the finest fluctuation. In the words of the University of California physicist Henry P. Stapp: 'An elementary particle is not an independently existing unanalyzable entity. It is, in essence, a set of relationships that reach outward to other things' (Davies 1984).

These deep relationships throughout creation – including connections between the objective world and the human mind – have long been understood and utilized in the tradition of Ayurveda. This branch of knowledge is known as *jyotish*. Trained Maharishi Jyotish experts use precise mathematical calculations to take into account important aspects of the environment including planets and stars (or 'cosmic counter-parts', as Maharishi calls them). These calculations are said to yield information about the health of an individual. Most importantly, this information can be used to predict health problems coming in the future. Maharishi frequently quotes the *Yoga Sutras*, a verse that says, *Heyam dukham anagatum* ('Avert the danger that has not yet come'). In MAV, *jyotish* is used to foresee dangers so proper preventive measures can be employed in time.

Maharishi Yagya

This modality is based on the same principle as primordial sound. Sequences of sound cognized by enlightened seers amount to a blueprint of the most basic laws of nature, 'DNA' for the universe. Physicists speak of the 'cosmic code', the mathematically describable laws of nature that structure creation. In Maharishi's explanation, the complex sound patterns in the Ṛk Veda and other central Vedic texts *are* this cosmic code. Information is carried by pronunciation, pitch, sequence, and rhythmic pattern. Every law of nature has its own unique pattern.

Maharishi Yagya involves *pandits* who perform particular sequences from these Vedic collections. The performance is said to enliven the particular laws of nature that correspond to the selections. This brings

balance to the environment as a whole. *Yagyas* can be performed for individuals, groups, nations, and the world as a whole. Choice of the particular *yagya* to be performed is often based on the calculations of *jyotish*, so that *yagyas* can be used to correct imbalances that have not yet manifested. The relative impact of the *yagya* is proportional to both the number of, and the purity of awareness of, the *pandits* who perform it.

Maharishi Sthapatya Veda

It may seem odd to include architecture as part of the Vedic Approach to Health, but doing so is prescient of the latest thinking in modern circles. Dwellings are being found to affect health in various ways today, from the positive effects of windows to the negative effects of indoor pollution. The Vedic Approach to Health, using the ancient architectural discipline of *Sthapatya Veda*, goes much further. To produce the maximum benefit to health, Maharishi Sthapatya Veda has numerous recommendations for architectural design.

One of its key concerns is orientation. According to Maharishi Sthapatya Veda, the orientation of houses, villages, towns and cities affects the inhabitants' health. This includes the position of the house on the land, the direction of the entrances, placement of rooms, and orientation of approaching and surrounding roads. Such positioning takes into account the internal positioning of rooms and community planning, as well as solar and lunar influences with reference to the Earth's magnetic poles and equator. (Research has in fact found that the human brain tissue contains crystals of magnetite, laying open the possibility that we are not insensitive to the effects of the earth's magnetic fields.)

A second concern is natural materials. Again, this is prescient: modern medicine is beginning to recognize the 'sick building syndrome'. Modern builders have been using increasingly toxic materials, including dyes, paints, and glues in wood products, carpets, and other elements of home construction. These materials can emit gases that are pathogenic. For example, formaldehyde from indoor pollution has been shown to cause mucous membrane irritation in large numbers of people, and may cause other health problems as well, some of them serious. There is also evidence that complex mixtures of volatile organic compounds in indoor air contribute to sensory irritation and possibly adversely influence the nervous system (Berglund et al 1996). To avoid such problems, Maharishi Sthapatya Veda gives detailed information about the use of natural building materials.

Natural ventilation is also a concern. In order to make air conditioning and heating more energy-efficient, modern builders have been insulating buildings far more tightly. The result is that toxic fumes become trapped inside. This can include not only toxins from man-made materials, but even naturally occurring pollutants, such as dust mites and by-products of insects and animals. *Sthapatya Veda* holds that the free flow of fresh air is essential for health, and has procedures for ensuring that this is provided.

A fourth concern is with natural settings. According to *Sthapatya Veda*, landscaping is not just decorative; it has an effect on health. Again, modern studies concur. Research has shown that patients whose hospital room windows looked out on a grove of deciduous trees had a shorter hospital stay and a more positive postsurgical recovery than a matched control group of patients whose windows looked out upon a building (Ulrich 1984). Research has suggested that human beings have evolved so as to have innate preferences for certain elements of landscape and habitat (Orians & Heerwagen 1992). These have interesting correspondences to *Sthapatya Veda* advice on healthful landscaping, but *Sthapatya Veda* adds other subtleties, for example, postulating that different types of landscape elements benefit different *doshas*.

By dealing with all of these and many other factors, *Sthapatya Veda* attempts to create dwellings that best promote health.

CONSCIOUSNESS

The TM-Sidhi program

In his Vedic Science, Maharishi offers additional technologies of consciousness. The most widely used is the TM-Sidhi program, a series of advanced meditation techniques. If the Transcendental Meditation technique is like diving to the deepest level of pure intelligence, the TM-Sidhi program is like underwater swimming – moving around *within* the field of pure intelligence. Established deep within, the mind entertains particular impulses of formulas (the Sanskrit word is *sutra*). At the ordinary active surface level of the mind's experience in everyday thinking, these *sutras* would produce no effect at all. But at the almost infinitely refined, subtle levels of the mind experienced as the mind transcends, each *sutra* gives a particular direction to pure consciousness. It stirs and enlivens that most basic level of natural law. Maharishi has described the process as follows:

The TM-Sidhi program trains the conscious mind to function in this field of pure consciousness. In the TM-Sidhi program one takes a sutra and it dissolves, and then another sutra and it dissolves. At that point when the first sutra has dissolved but the second one has not yet emerged is the experience of the self-referral state of consciousness. In this state the previous sutra is transforming itself into the next. The gap between the two sutras is a self-referral state of awareness, but it has that dynamism of one transforming into the other ... Physicists call this the self-interacting quality of the unified field. Those who practice the TM-Sidhi program experience that self-interacting quality as one value transforms itself into another value. (Maharishi Mahesh Yogi 1986).

When the mind is trapped in superficial awareness of the surface appearance of the world, it sees only objects and action. This limited experience is all that can be metabolized by the body. Transcendental Meditation and the TM-Sidhi program expand this experience. The mind experiences not only objects, but also the subject – the deepest level of its own nature. It knows not only action, but also silence – the unbounded consciousness at the basis of activity. The outward stroke of the mind, experiencing the world created by natural law, is balanced by an inward stroke, experiencing the *source* of natural law. MAV maintains that this enriched experience balances the *doshas*, and thereby prevents disease before it can arise. The voluminous research we saw on the health effects of Transcendental Meditation, including reduced health-care utilization, supports this conclusion.

The TM-Sidhi program has given rise to another remarkable field of research, involving the largest possible application of MAV – on society as a whole. We will conclude this chapter by discussing it.

Collective health

At first glance, it might seem that violent crime and war fall outside the purview of the health-care provider. Yet a visit to a war zone – a real war zone, or the high-crime areas referred to by that term – would convince one that these are more than sociological concerns. It is not only the toll of mortality and bodily injuries; violent situations also profoundly affect the psychologies of survivors or of those trapped in them, in ways that certainly affect both mental and physical health. They can even affect the health of those on the periphery, as people used to dealing with the tensions of urban life may experience.

The most far-reaching of all MAV programs address these large-scale illnesses of society. A famous phrase from the *Yoga Sutras* reads, *Tat sannidhau vairatyagah* ('In the vicinity of the settled mind, hostile tendencies fall away'). Now, more than 40 separate scientific studies have shown that meditation experts can create a statistically measurable influence of harmony and peace in their environment. This research supports strongly the idea that meditation can change the world around us.

The studies show that when a sufficient percentage of the population practices TM, or whenever a sufficient number of experts in Transcendental Meditation and the TM-Sidhi program practice their programs together, crime decreases, traffic accidents go down, and open warfare (if it is present) declines.

The reason scientists began to look at statistics of this sort was a theoretical prediction: in 1960, Maharishi had predicted that a small percentage of a population practicing Transcendental Meditation would be sufficient to influence the trends of life in their society (for this reason researchers have named this phenomenon 'the Maharishi Effect'). An unpublished study (1977) carried out by MIU researchers Candace Borland and Garland Landrith III found that, in cities with at least 1% of their populations practicing the TM program, the crime rate dropped compared to control cities. This study was later extended by Landrith along with Michael Dillbeck and Orme-Johnson (Dillbeck et al 1981), and became the first published study on the subject. In this later study, the experimental group consisted of all cities in the United States with populations larger than 10 000 and in which at least 1% of the

population had learned the TM technique by the end of 1972. The selection of carefully matched control cities was supervised by an independent investigator from another university, and yielded 24 control and 24 experimental cities. The researchers took their crime rate data from the *Uniform Crime Reports*, published by the US Department of Justice.

The results bore out the theory. Compared to the crime rate in the control cities, crime rates in the '1%' cities fell significantly after the 1% threshold had been reached, and stayed lower for the five subsequent years studied. The changes could not be explained by changes in other demographic factors that might be related to crime, such as percentage of families with incomes below the poverty level, percentage of people in the age ranges of 15 to 29 years, population density, median years of education, population turnover, unemployment rate, and per capita income. The findings were published in the peer-reviewed *Journal of Crime and Justice*.

At first, it might seem impossible that a group of meditators, who seem to have no interactions with the criminals or to be criminals themselves (Dillbeck et al 1988, pp 484–485), could affect the criminal tendencies of others without any physical or verbal interaction at all. However, this follows naturally if consciousness is, like every other aspect of nature, an unbounded field, as we suggested in Chapter 2. Any field in nature can support radiating waves that create field effects and action at a distance. A television station can radiate invisible, non-material waves through the underlying electromagnetic field. The result is a TV picture in your living room. Thus the '1%' research could be said to provide evidence that consciousness can have field-like effects.

The TM-Sidhi program, which we discussed in our last section, was introduced in the mid-1970s; because it involves a more powerful enlivenment of pure consciousness, it was predicted to have a much more powerful sociological effect. Moreover, since the first study in 1977, increasingly sophisticated research methods have become available, such as causal and time-series analysis, to better control for other possible factors that might have caused the outcomes. These advanced methods have never located any hidden or alternative variables. The 'field effect' that has emerged from such studies is that a group of TM-Sidhi practitioners – equal to about the square root of 1% of a population – when practicing their techniques together, can dramatically reduce crime, war deaths, and other negative factors not only in their own cities, but far away, even as much as halfway around the world.

One significant study of this sort took place in Israel in 1983. A group of TM and TM-Sidhi practitioners met daily in Jerusalem to practice their techniques together in a group. The group size fluctuated from day to day, but when it reached certain critical thresholds, statistics showed measurable changes for the entire population of Jerusalem and of Israel as a whole. This group size amounted to the square root of 1% of the population of the city or the country. Whenever the group size reached these thresholds, city and national life improved dramatically. Sufficient group size was associated with reduced automobile accidents, fires, and crime. The correlations were high. Controlling for other variables showed that the correlations were not likely to be coincidences.

To further test the theory, the researchers (who were from Harvard and Maharishi International University) examined what happened to the Lebanon war on the days when the group size reached a larger threshold – one predicted to influence that neighboring country. They analyzed this by comparing the daily size of the group with the daily number of war deaths and the intensity of fighting in Lebanon (as measured by a standard 'content analysis' measure applied to newspapers). The results were dramatic. Every time the group size reached threshold, the war deaths and intensity decreased. The scientists had never in their careers seen so high a statistical correlation.

This study was published in the *Journal of Conflict Resolution* (Orme-Johnson et al 1988). The journal's editor, Professor Raymond Russ of the University of Maine, said: 'The hypothesis definitely raised some eyebrows among our reviewers. But the statistical work was sound. The numbers were there... where you can statistically control for as many variables as these studies do, it makes the results more convincing' (personal communication, 1992).

The Jerusalem group was, unfortunately, not maintained. But other groups have been convened in other areas, and published studies on their effects have extended the findings. Over two dozen studies of such coherence-creating groups have indicated that dis-

tance did not mediate their effects, though population size did. If the TM-Sidhi group was large enough, its effect could, according to the theory, be felt throughout a certain size of population, no matter how spread out that population was geographically. Assemblies of TM-Sidhi experts in Iowa (winter 1983 and summer 1984), Yugoslavia (spring 1984), the Netherlands (winter 1984), and Washington, D.C., (summer 1985) all had groups large enough (containing between 2500 and 7000 people) to affect the population of Lebanon, according to John Davies, now of the University of Maryland Center for the Study of Peace and Conflict Resolution. Davies did a time-series analysis using independently derived statistics, and found on average a 66% increase in cooperation between antagonists in the Lebanese war, a 48% reduction in armed conflict, a 71% reduction in war deaths, and a 68% reduction in war injuries. Analyzing the data as a whole, in order to filter out statistical 'noise', Davies found that the probability of these results having happened by chance was less than 1 in 10 million trillion (Davies 1988).

One finding in several studies (including the above two) was that the largest effect on Lebanon came not from the *nearest* group, the one in Lebanon itself in spring 1984, but, rather, from the *largest* group – 7000 people, a group large enough, by the theory of the 'field effect', to affect the entire world. This group had convened in Fairfield, Iowa, in winter 1983. This highlighted a central question: how could groups of people in the United States or the Netherlands have such a big effect on a population in the Middle East? And why should the particular threshold involved – the square root of 1% of the population – be effective?

We return to the idea of a 'field effect'. Consider the surface of a pond. Start a wave, and all the corks bob even though you didn't hit them directly. The wave is propagated across the surface of the pond, the 'field'. Coherent field effects are found in many physical systems. For example, laser light, which is used in CD players but can also cut through metals, is just ordinary light made coherent through a field effect. It results when the light particles (photons), which in usual light move in many different directions, make a *phase transition* and begin to move together perfectly coherently. To turn ordinary light into laser light all that is needed is for a few light particles – about the square root of 1% of the total population of photons – to become coherent together. (At these subtle levels of nature, the effect of coherent elements is proportionate to the *square* of their number.) Their effect is carried to the rest of the light particles through the quantum *field* of light – each light particle is a wave on that underlying field. Physics calls this phenomenon 'super radiance'. Thus, a very small fraction of individual units in a system can have a huge effect on the system as a whole.

Nature often repeats basic patterns in disparate systems. Davies and other researchers have found that coherence in a human population is produced by the same proportion as in a physical system, the square root of 1% of the individuals, becoming coherent within themselves. What kind of field would carry coherence through a group of people? For a variety of reasons, Dr John Hagelin argues that it could not be any of the four known force fields of nature – electromagnetism, gravity, strong interactions and weak interactions. The human brain does produce electromagnetic effects and is influenced by them, but these are far too small to be able to affect large numbers of other people. Hagelin (1987) maintains that it could only be mediated through the unified field, which has the property of infinite correlation – an effect anywhere is felt everywhere. It will not decrease owing to distance, nor will it be delayed in farther-away places, because the unified field exists at a level of nature (called the Planck scale) which is deeper than space or time.

The American philosopher William James said that on the surface we seem as separate from each other as islands in the sea, but, like islands, we are connected at the ocean floor – which he called, in our case, 'a continuum of cosmic consciousness'. That continuum of consciousness is how Vedic Science has traditionally described what physics calls the unified field: as the field of pure consciousness. This is why a group of people becoming orderly, peaceful, and blissful in their own consciousness – transcending to the level of pure consciousness – could create a positive, coherent influence in other people. For this 'super radiance' effect, the relevant field is consciousness, and the 'waves on the field' are minds. If enough people are creating coherence in the field, the effect could be felt as far away from Iowa as Lebanon.

Other studies are consistent with the above effect.

Such studies have considered negative indicators like rates of suicide, accidents, and infectious diseases (as well as crime) and positive indicators like the number of patent applications. The studies have focused on various levels of social organization, including cities (Dillbeck et al 1988), states, countries, and, in one study conducted in winter 1983, the world as a whole. They have been conducted in a number of different countries, including India, the Philippines, the Netherlands, Zimbabwe, and many others, which verifies the universality of the effect across cultural lines. They continue to verify the hypothesis; none so far have failed to confirm it.

We have compared a human life to a tree, and said that transcendental consciousness, the state experienced in TM, waters the root so that the whole tree benefits. To extend this analogy, when enough people water their own root, the water table under the whole forest rises so that the whole forest becomes greener – that is, more harmonious, happy, and peaceful.

In a speech delivered to the World Bank in Washington, D.C., Dr Kurleigh D. King, the former Secretary-General of the Caribbean Economic Community and Governor of the Central Bank of Barbados, pointed out that although MAV's theory of collective consciousness is unlike anything we are used to, it is now more thoroughly researched and documented than any other approach to world peace. Some laudable attempts are being made by various physicians to address the problems of society. This research suggests a particularly effective and profound contribution that the physician can make – and through a means that also makes profound contributions to patients' individual health.

CONCLUSION

As stated at the outset of this book, we do not dismiss modern medicine and its achievements; but we must again point out that it does not consider all the factors that influence health, and that this lack of consideration can cause serious problems. Many important factors are not considered at all in the current system. This book has introduced a number of such areas – areas that Maharishi's Vedic Approach to Health considers in detail, from consciousness through the many elements considered above.

As we have seen throughout the book, promising research has validated the Maharishi Vedic Approach, and extensive clinical experience worldwide has borne it out. Future research and clinical experience with MAV will continue to make important contributions to medical practice and scientific understanding.

We have stated that the basic model on which modern medicine is based is inadequate. We suggest that research and experience in MAV will give rise to a new medical paradigm, with great potential for improving human health. We have called this 'the consciousness model'. It is hoped that this book has given some insight into our belief that a truly satisfactory medical model must begin at the foundation of human experience.

REFERENCES

Berglund B, Brunekreef B, Knoeppel H et al 1996 Effects of indoor air pollution on human health. Reprint 10, EUR 14086EN. Office for Official Publications of the European Community, Luxembourg

Bruya M A, Severtsen B 1984 Evaluating the effects of music on electroencephalogram patterns of normal subjects. Journal of Neurosurgical Nursing 16(2):96–100

Chou K-C 1983 Identification of low-frequency modes in protein molecules. Biochemistry Journal 209:573–580

Chou K-C 1984 Low-frequency vibrations of DNA molecules. Biochemistry Journal 221:27–31

Cook J D 1981 The therapeutic use of music: a literature review. Nursing Forum 20(3): 252–266

Cook J D 1986 Music as an intervention in the oncology setting. Cancer Nursing 9(1): 23–28

Davies P 1984 Superforce: the search for a grand unified theory of nature. Touchstone, Simon & Schuster, New York, p. 49

Davies J 1988 Alleviating political violence through enhancing coherence in collective consciousness: impact assessment analysis of the Lebanon war. Dissertation Abstracts International 49(8):2381(A)

Dillbeck M C, Landrith G S, Orme-Johnson D W 1981 The Transcendental Meditation program and crime rate change in a sample of 48 cities. Journal of Crime and Justice 4:25–45

Dillbeck M C, Banus C B, Polanzi G, Landrith G 1988 Test of a field model of consciousness and social change: the Transcendental Meditation and TM-Sidhi program and decreased urban crime. Journal of Mind and Behavior 9:457–486

Hagelin J 1987 Is consciousness the unified field? A field theorist's perspective. Modern Science and Vedic Science, 1:29–87

Karplus M, McCammon J A 1986 The dynamics of proteins. Scientific American 254(4):42–51

Lawrence J B, Singer R H, Marselle L M 1989 Highly localized tracks of specific transcripts within interphase nuclei visualized by in situ hybridization. Cell 57:493–502

McClelland D C 1979 Music in the operating room. Journal of the Association of Operating Room Nurses 29(2):252–260

Maharishi Mahesh Yogi 1986 Life supported by natural law. Age of Enlightenment, Washington DC p 25

Maharishi Mahesh Yogi 1995 Maharishi's Vedic Approach to Health. Maharishi Vedic University, Vlodrop, Netherlands

Mohler J L, Partin A W, Coffey D S 1987 Prediction of metastatic potential by a new grading system of cell motility: validation in the Dunning R-3327 prostatic adenocarcinoma model. Journal of Urology 138:168

Munro S, Mount B 1978 Music therapy in palliative care. Canadian Medical Association Journal 119:1029–1034

Myrdal S E, Auersperg N 1986 An agent or agents produced by virus-transformed cells cause unregulated ruffling in untransformed cells. Journal of Cell Biology 102:1224–1229

Nader T 1995 Human physiology: expression of Veda and the Vedic literature. Maharishi Vedic University Press, Vlodrop, Netherlands

Orians G H, Heerwagen J H 1992 Evolved responses to landscapes. In: Barkow J H, Cosmides L, Tooby J (eds) The adapted mind. Oxford University Press, New York, pp 555–580

Orme-Johnson D, Alexander C N, Davies J L, Chandler H M, Larimore W E 1988 International peace project in the Middle East: the effects of the Maharishi Technology of the Unified Field. Journal of Conflict Resolution 32:776–812

O'Sullivan R J 1991 A musical road to recovery: music in intensive care. Intensive Care Nursing 7:160–163

Owens M K, Ehrenreich D 1991 Literature review of nonpharmacologic methods for the treatment of chronic pain. Holistic Nursing Practice 6(1):24–31

Partin A W, Isaacs J T, Treiger B, Coffey D S 1988 Early cell motility changes associated with an increase in metastatic ability in rat prostatic cancer cells transfected with the v-harvey-ras oncogene. Cancer Research 48:6050–6053

Pienta K J, Coffey D S 1991 Cellular harmonic information transfer through a tissue tensegrity-matrix system. Medical Hypotheses 34:88–95

Sharma H M, Alexander C N 1996 Maharishi Ayurveda: research review. Part 2: Maharishi Ayurveda herbal food supplements and additional strategies. Complementary Medicine International 3(2):17–28

Sharma H M, Kauffman E M, Stephens R E 1996 Effect of different sounds on growth of human cancer cell lines in vitro. Alternative Therapies in Clinical Practice 3(4):25–32

Sitter A J, Reczek C M, Terner J 1985 Observance of the $Fe^{IV} = 0$ stretching vibration of ferryl myoglobin by resonance Raman spectroscopy. Biochimica Biophysica Acta 828: 229–235

Ulrich R 1984 Views through a window may influence recovery from surgery. Science 224:420–421

Xing Y, Lawrence J B 1989 Highly localized tracks of nuclear RNA are not disrupted by nuclear matrix isolation procedures. Journal of Cell Biology 109:315a (abstract)

Appendices

Appendix 1

Pronunciation guide

We have not included all Sanskrit words used in this book, but only those whose pronunciations might be difficult to work out without the application of the following rules.

In two-syllable words, the first syllable is accented. For longer words, see individual entries.

The vowel represented by 'a' is the so-called *schwa*; it rhymes with 'huh'.

The vowel represented by 'o' rhymes with dough, sew, toe, and row.

The vowel represented by 'ā' is the long 'a' found in the formula tra-la-la.

The vowel represented by 'ū' is a long u, as in 'cool'.

The vowel represented by 'u' is the short u found in 'push' (*except* at the end of words, where it sounds more like the long 'u'.

The vowel represented by 'ay' (usually transliterated by the letter e) rhymes with day.

The vowel represented by 'i' is what is found in the word 'pin'.

The vowel represented by 'ī' is what is found in 'he' or 'she'.

abhyanga	a-BHYANG-ga
ahamkara	a han-Kā-ra
alochaka	a-LO-cha-ka
apana	a-Pā-na
buddhi	BUD-dhī
chhandas	CHHAN-das
devata	DAY-va-tā
dhatu	DHā-tu
Kapha	KA-fa
lavana	LA-va-na
madhura	MA-dhu-ra
mahabhutas	ma-hā-BHŪ-tas
mamsa	MāM-sa
meda	MAY-da
mrdhu	MRI-dhu
pachaka	Pā-cha-ka
panchakarma	pan-cha-KAR-ma
pandit	PAN-dit ('pan' rhymes with 'pun')
pragya-aparadh	pragyāparādh
prakriti	PRA-kri-ti
ranjaka	RAN-ja-ka
rasayana	ra-Sā-ya-na
sadhaka	Sā-dha-ka
samana	sa-Mā-na
samhita	SANG-hi-tā (Note: the first syllable is pronounced 'sung')
sasneha	sa-SNAY-ha
shita	SHĪ-ta
snehana	SNAY-ha-na
swedana	SWAY-da-na

tanmatra	tan-MA-tra ('tan' rhymes with 'pun')	veda	VAY-da
tikshna	TIKSH-na	virya	VIR-ya
udana	u-Dā-na	vishada	vi-SHā-da
Vata	Vā-ta	vyana	VYā-na
Vayu	Vā-yu		

Appendix 2

Resources

This book presents a comprehensive natural health care system, which includes the underlying theoretical basis and research conducted on various modalities of this health care system. No one, however, should attempt to treat an illness or disorder simply on this basis. If there is an illness, a physician should be consulted.

To locate a physician in your area trained in Maharishi Ayur-Veda, or for information on training programs in the different aspects of Maharishi Ayur-Veda:

USA

Maharishi Ayur-Veda University, PO Box 8196, Chicago, IL 60680-8196, USA

Tel: 1 800 843 8332
      1 800 888 5797

UK

Maharishi Ayur-Veda College of Natural Medicine, Mentmore Towers, Mentmore, Bucks LU7 0QH, UK

Tel: 44 1296 661726

Europe

Maharishi Vedic University, Department of Health Care, Kloosterweg 36, 6301 WK Valkenburg, The Netherlands

Tel: 31 43 60 14 568
Fax: 31 43 60 13 262

India

Maharishi Mahesh Yogi Vedic Vishwa Vidyalaya, 871 Napier Town, Jabalpur, Madhya Pradesh 482001, India

Tel: 91 761 410325
Fax: 91 761 315722

Australia

Maharishi Vedic University, 345 Grimshaw Road, Bundoora, Victoria 3083, Australia

Tel: 61 3 9467 4633
Fax: 61 3 9467 4688

Maharishi Ayur-Veda Health Centres

A list of the major health centers which provide the Maharishi Ayur-Veda technologies discussed in this book follows:

USA

The Raj, Maharishi Ayur-Veda Health Center, 1734 Jasmine Avenue, Fairfield, IA 52556, USA

Tel: 800 248 9050
 515 472 9580
Fax: 515 472 2496

Maharishi Ayur-Veda Health Center, 679 George Hill Road, Lancaster, MA 01523, USA

Tel: 508 365 4549
Fax: 508 368 7557

Maharishi Ayur-Veda Health Center, 17308 Sunset Boulevard, Pacific Palisades, CA 90270, USA

Tel: 310 454 5531
Fax: 310 454 7841

Maharishi Ayur-Veda Health Center, 4910 Massachusetts Avenue NW, Suite 315, Washington, DC 20016, USA

Tel: 202 244 2700
Fax: 202 244 7695

UK

Maharishi Ayur-Veda Health Centre, The Golden Dome, Woodley Park, Skelmersdale, Lancs WN8 6UQ, United Kingdom

Tel: 44 1695 51008

Maharishi Ayur-Veda Health Centre, 24 Linhope Street, London NW1 6HT, United Kingdom

Tel: 44 171 724 6267

Maharishi Ayur-Veda Health Centre, Roydon Hall, Seven Mile Lane, East Peckham, Tonbridge, Kent TN12 5NH, United Kingdom

Tel: 44 1622 812121

Europe

Maharishi Vedic University, Department of Health Care, Kloosterweg 36, 6301 WK Valkenburg, The Netherlands

Tel: 31 43 60 14 568
Fax: 31 43 60 13 262

Maharishi Ayur-Veda Gesundheitszentrum, Parkschlösschen Bad Wildstein, Wildbadstr. 201, 56841 Traben-Trarbach, Germany

Tel: 49 6541 7050
Fax: 49 6541 705 120

Maharishi Ayur-Veda Gesundheits- und Seminarzentrum, Am Robert Kampe Sprudel, Postfach 13 30, 56120 Bad Ems, Germany

Tel: 49 2603 94070
Fax: 49 2603 3122

Maharishi Ayur-Veda Gesundheitszentrum, Pilgerheim, 6377 Seelisberg, Switzerland

Tel: 41 41 820 57 50
Fax: 41 41 820 52 86

India

Maharishi Ayurveda Arogyadham (Khosla Hospital), Block – B, Pocket – P, Shalimar Bagh (West), Delhi – 110 052, India

Tel: 91 11 741 2069
Fax: 91 11 683 6682

For information on Maharishi Ayur-Veda herbal food supplements

USA

Maharishi Ayur-Veda Products International, Inc., P.O. Box 49667, Colorado Springs, CO 80949–9667, USA

Tel: 1 800 255 8332
Fax: 719 260 7400

Canada

Maharishi Ayur-Veda Products, P.O. Box 9402, 40 Chemin Cochrane, Compton, Quebec J0B 1L0, Canada

Tel: 1 800 461 9685
Fax: 819 835 9590

UK

Maharishi Ayur-Veda Products, Peel House, Peel Road, West Pimbo, Skelmersdale, Lancashire WN8 9PT, UK

Tel: 44 1695 51015
Fax: 44 1695 50917

Europe

Maharishi Technology Corporation BV, Tussen de Bruggen 10, 6063 NA Vlodrop, The Netherlands

Tel: 31 475 404060
Fax: 31 475 404055

India

Maharishi Ayurveda Corporation Ltd., A-14, Mohan Co-op. Industrial Estate, Mathura Road, New Delhi - 110 044, India

Tel: 91 11 694 6501
 91 11 694 6502
 91 11 694 6503
 91 11 694 6504
Fax: 91 11 683 6682

Australia

Maharishi Ayur-Veda Products, PO Box 81, Bundoora, Victoria 3083, Australia

Tel: 61 3 9467 4633
Fax: 61 3 9467 4688

New Zealand

MAP New Zealand, 9 Adam Street, Greenlane, Auckland, New Zealand

Tel: 64 9 524 5883
Fax: 64 9 524 5430

Index